ASSESSMENT AND TREATMENT OF SCHOOL-AGE LANGUAGE DISORDERS

A RESOURCE MANUAL

Rita C. Naremore, Ph.D.

Ann E. Densmore, M.A.

Department of Speech and Hearing Sciences
Indiana University, Bloomington, Indiana

Deborah R. Harman, M.A.T.

Country School Corporation
Nashville, Indiana

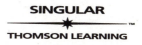

SINGULAR

™

THOMSON LEARNING

Australia Canada Mexico Singapore Spain United Kingdom United States

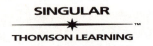

SINGULAR

™

THOMSON LEARNING

Assessment and Treatment of School-Age Language Disorders: A Resource Manual
by Rita C. Naremore,, Ph.D., Anne E. Densmore, M.A., and Deborah R. Harman, M.A.T.

Business Unit Director:
William Brotmiller

Acquisitions Editor:
Marie Linville

Editorial Assistant:
Kristin Banach

Executive Marketing Manager:
Dawn Gerrain

Channel Manager:
Tara Carter

Executive Production Editor:
Karen Leet

Production Editor:
Sandy Doyle

Library of Congress Cataloging-in-Publication Data
Naremore, Rita C.
Assessment and treatment for school-age language disorders: a resource manual / Rita C. Naremore, Ann E. Densmore, Deborah R. Harman.
    p. ; cm.
Includes bibilographical references and index.
ISBN 0-7693-0056-1 (pbk. : alk. paper)
1. Language disorders—Handbooks, manuals, etc. 2. Language disorders in children—Handbooks, manuals, etc. 3. Speech disorders in children—Handbooks,
manuals, etc. I. Densmore, Ann E. II. Harman, Deborah R. III. Title.
[DNLM: 1. Language Disorders—diagnosis—Child—Resource Guides. 2. Language Disorders—therapy—Child—Resource Guides. WL 39 N225a 2001]
RJ496.L35 N37 2001
618.92'855—dc21   00-30051

NOTICE TO THE READER

ASSESSMENT AND TREATMENT OF SCHOOL-AGE LANGUAGE DISORDERS

A RESOURCE MANUAL

Contents

PART II: NARRATIVE

PART III: ADVANCED LITERACY SKILLS

Preface

About This Book

> This is a book of practical, useful, reality-based assessment tools and intervention ideas designed to help practicing speech-language pathologists conduct assessment and treatment with children's phonological awareness, narrative, and advanced literacy skills. The assessment and intervention ideas included in this book are all designed to help practicing clinicians move toward educationally relevant goals and objectives.

This book is intended to be first and foremost a practical compendium of assessment instruments and intervention ideas. It is designed for the school speech-language pathologist who is concerned with making language assessment and intervention relevant to the academic success of children with language impairments. It is based on two convictions that we hold strongly:

1. Children with language problems *can* develop the language they need to succeed in school if we focus our assessment and intervention practices on the language skills they need for academic success.

2. The school speech-language pathologist is an educator, a person whose expertise should be devoted toward helping children with communication impairments succeed in the academic environment of the school.

Unique Features

This manual focuses on three areas of language where language impaired children in elementary school need particular help: phonological awareness, narrative skills, and advanced literacy skills.

- Nonstandardized, criterion-based assessment tasks are provided for use in determining a child's strengths and weaknesses in language areas that are critical to academic success. Research data are provided, demonstrating how we constructed our own pass-fail criteria for these tasks.

The phonological awareness section contains a rhyming task designed to be used for kindergarten and early first grade children, together with a 70-item phonological awareness task that assesses sound isolation, blending, and segmentation. The narrative skills section explains how to use story retelling as an assessment technique, and provides scoring sheets for stories appropriate for kindergarten, first, and second grade children. The advanced literacy skills section contains a task that can be used to evaluate a child's ability to find main idea at various levels of difficulty ranging from pictures to short paragraphs, as well as ideas for assessing children's inferencing abilities.

- Sample intervention activities are provided in each area, and include examples of materials that can be duplicated. We discuss how to reason from test results to goals, and sample goals and objectives, along with sample lesson plans in each area, are included. These are intended to provide a framework onto which clinicians can graft activities and materials appropriate for the individual children with whom they are working.
- This manual will be particularly useful for school practitioners attempting to meet the IDEA requirements for educationally relevant goals developed collaboratively. The sample goals and objectives found in this manual were developed by one school speech-language pathologist in collaboration with special educators and regular classroom teachers in her school. They are designed to fit with the language arts curriculum found in most early elementary school classrooms.

Acknowledgments

We are grateful to Michael, who did not arrive until Debbie had almost finished her part of the manuscript, and to Stephanie, who came along just in time to save Rita's sanity, and to the classroom teachers who taught Ann more than she ever wanted to know about collaboration. Most of all, we want to acknowledge the graduate students who have participated in the Language to Learn program for the past 5 years. They helped us test more than 400 children, and developed intervention ideas we might never have thought of, left to ourselves. They learned along with us about the fun, the frustrations, and the rewards of working with children in the schools.

INTRODUCTION

Making Language Assessment and Intervention Academically Relevant

What aspects of language are the foci for academically relevant assessment and intervention?

Research investigating the academic achievement of children with communication impairments has shown repeatedly that these children encounter significant difficulties in school. They are particularly at risk for failure to learn to read and to learn to express their ideas in writing (Catts & Kamhi, 1998; Wallach & Butler, 1994). Children who lack basic literacy are unable to acquire the new knowledge presented to them in the classroom. They are unable to use writing to take notes or to preserve their ideas for later use. Further research has demonstrated the interaction of a child's language abilities with the acquisition and use of literacy skills in school (Bishop & Adams, 1990; Catts, 1993; Fazio, Naremore, & Connell, 1996; Liles, Duffy, Merritt, & Purcell, 1995). As more is learned about the language base for academic success, clinicians understand more about what children with communication impairments need.

- A growing body of research evidence suggests that working with a child's phonological awareness abilities strengthens the child's ability to decode printed words (Ball & Blachman, 1991; Liberman & Shankweiler, 1985; Lundberg, Frost, & Petersen, 1988; Mann, 1993). Children with language impairments are particularly at risk for difficulties with phonological awareness, and in need of training beyond that provided in the typical classroom (Blachman, Ball, Black, & Tange, 1994; Catts, 1993; Kamhi & Catts, 1986).
- Other evidence suggests that a child's ability to structure oral narratives is related to the child's reading comprehension, as well as the ability to

1

structure written narratives (Anderson, 1994; Fazio et al., 1996; Hansen, 1978; Klecan-Aker & Caraway, 1997; Westby, 1998). Children with language impairments seem to have particular difficulty forming and using narrative frameworks to understand and compose narratives and direct teaching can help them (Gillam, McFadden, & van Kleek, 1995; Graham, MacArthur, Schwartz, & Voth, 1992; Palinscar & Brown, 1984; Sawyer, Graham, & Harris, 1992).

- As children progress through school, they must move from a focus on acquiring literacy to a focus on using literacy to acquire and communicate about increasingly complex ideas and concepts. Advanced literacy skills, such as finding the main idea of a text or making appropriate inferences based on a text, become critical to the child's learning. These skills are particularly difficult for children with language impairment, and the instruction provided in the general classroom does not generally allow the repeated practice and slower presentation of new information needed by these children (Roller & Schreiner, 1985; Scott; 1989; Wallach, 1990; Wong, 1982). Speech-language pathologists who are expert at task analysis can break down these tasks for both the child and the teacher and can help by assessing a child's level of ability and by providing appropriate intervention activities designed to help a child develop advanced literacy skills.

How can the information in this book be used?

Using the Information for Assessment Purposes

A full-range assessment of a child's language can have several purposes, including to:

- Determine whether the child's language use is within normal limits,
- Specify areas of relative strength and weakness, and
- Provide information needed to plan appropriate intervention.

Assessment of the language base for academic success is particularly important for the latter two purposes. The environment in which a school-aged child must function is, after all, the classroom. We need to determine whether a child has the language abilities needed to function in that environment and, if not, the level at which appropriate intervention should begin. Assessment tasks that simply indicate what a child cannot do are not useful for planning intervention. We need assessment tasks that enable us to simplify the level at which a child is asked to perform until we find a level at which the child can succeed. This is what we have attempted to do with the assessment tools provided in this book. For example, if a child cannot isolate the initial sound in words, can the child detect rhymes? If not, can the child break words into syllables? Syllabification and rhyme detection developmentally precede sound isolation and seem to form the basis for that skill. If a child cannot retell a complete episode from a multi-episode story, can the child consistently retell parts of the episodes? If not, can the child fill in parts of the episodes if the examiner provides the other parts? The point is to systematically simplify an assessment task to determine the level at which a child can succeed, and also to allow sensible goals and objectives to be determined based on increasingly difficult levels of the target skill.

How are the assessment instruments in this book different from others?

Given the inadequacies of most of the standardized tests used to assess children's language, one might ask why clinicians continue to use them. There is one simple answer: standardized tests provide norms. They give us a picture of how children at various ages performed on the test and allow us to compare the performance of an individual child against these norms to determine whether his or her performance is like that of other children in the same age range. There are many problems with this procedure, but addressing these problems is not our focus here. All of the assessment instruments we talk about in this book are nonstandardized, criterion-referenced measures. The question at issue here is how to use these nonstandardized assessment instruments to help clinicians decide whether a given child should receive intervention for some aspect of language. If a 7-year-old child cannot isolate the beginning sound in words, does this mean intervention for phonological awareness is needed? If a first grader cannot retell an episodic story while looking at pictures, does this mean the child needs help in forming and using a story framework? How can these questions be answered without norms?

Assessment instruments may be *norm-referenced*, meaning that a child's performance is compared with that of other children, or they may be *criterion-referenced*, meaning that a child's score is evaluated in terms of some preset level of performance that is viewed as adequate or appropriate for the child's grade level.

1. Collecting Local Norms

In the face of these and similar questions, two approaches can be taken. The first is often referred to as "collecting local norms." To collect local norms for a particular task, it is necessary to test at least 100 children in the relevant grade or at the relevant age level (say, first graders or children between 8 and 10 years old). This group should include children who are performing across the continuum for their age or grade. In other words, if first graders are the target group, some of the children should be good readers, some average, and some poor or nonreaders. It is not necessary to test all the children at one time, but it might be important to test them at about the same point in the school year, depending on what skill is being assessed. For example, many beginning first graders are unable to blend sounds to make a word. That is, given the individual sounds in a word one sound at a time, they cannot put the individual sounds together and come up with a word. By the end of first grade, however, many children are able to do this, especially with familiar words. If local norms were being gathered for first grade children on a phonological awareness task over, say, a 3-year period, it would be important to test all the children at the same point in the academic year and to note the testing time when referring to these norms. Once a sufficient number of children in a given school system have been tested, means and standard deviations can be calculated for the scores and local criteria can be determined for including children in training. When we refer to local norms in this book, we report the number of children tested, the point in the academic year when they were tested, and our criterion score (which was usually one standard deviation below the mean for the group).

A related procedure that may be followed is less formal and less rigorous. It might be called "using average sampling." If a clinician needs to find out if a child's performance on a particular language task is below average for a particular class of children, the classroom teacher might be asked to name five or six children in the class who are average performers. The clinician might then test these children and, if their scores on the language measure seem to cluster (that is, if they are fairly consistent with one another), then a range of "average scores" for that classroom can be identified. The performance of the target child can then be compared with this range and may be characterized as "slightly below the average range" or "well below the average range" for the classroom. This procedure should not be referred to as "collecting local norms," nor should the test scores of the "average" children necessarily be carried over from one school to another. A small set of scores is more likely than a larger set to be influenced by the classroom practices of individual teachers or the approaches taken in particular curriculum materials. This "average sampling" approach is intended only to give a clinician a way to talk with parents or teachers about a child's performance in terms of the performance of a specific peer group. It can be justified only by the fact that both educators and parents tend to judge a child's language performance in terms of a set of expectations based largely on their experience with other children in the same grade or at the same age. A child who is regarded as well below average for his or her classroom in school A may be only slightly below average in school B. Such relative placement in a classroom continuum will certainly play a role in whether the child is referred for assessment and whether the child is able to keep up with the other children in the classroom.

2. Criterion-Referenced Testing

Using test norms, whether for formally standardized tests or from local populations, involves comparing a child's performance with the performance of other children. There is an alternative way of viewing a child's performance. By using research data and conferring with teachers about the demands of the classroom, one can determine a level of performance on a given measure that is adequate for a child in a particular grade. To give an example of what we mean, consider the criterion we use to judge whether a child's story retelling performance is adequate. Research (Fazio et al., 1996) has indicated that children who could not retell at least 50% of the episodes in a simple episodic story were at risk for academic failure. For this reason, we set our "pass/fail" cutoff for the story-retelling task at this level. *A child who cannot retell at least 50% of the episodes is not performing at a level likely to ensure academic success.* Notice that we do not say "a child who cannot retell at least 50% of the episodes is below average." A statement like that can only be made if you are comparing a given child's score with the scores of a group of other children. We are not doing that. We are evaluating the child's score in terms of whether it meets a level of performance known to be appropriate on a particular task. As we discuss specific assessment instruments throughout the book, we provide the criteria we used to determine whether a child's performance was adequate.

How do norm-referenced and criterion-referenced tests differ?

For a complete discussion of this, you might want to refer to McCauley (1996). Her discussion is briefly summarized:

- The purpose of norm-referenced tests is to rank children in comparison with one another. The purpose of criterion-referenced tests is to distinguish levels of performance.
- Norm-referenced tests typically cover a broad range of content. Criterion-referenced tests are designed to cover a specific domain in depth.
- In developing a norm-referenced test, we attempt to find items that will distinguish between children who perform well and those who perform poorly. In developing a criterion-referenced test, clinicians attempt to find items to adequately sample the content domain.
- Performance on norm-referenced tests is summarized using percentiles or standard scores. Performance on criterion-referenced tests is summarized using raw scores.
- The purpose of norm-referenced tests is to rank children in comparison with one another. The purpose of criterion-referenced tests is to distinguish levels of performance.

Using the Information for Intervention

This information can also be used for intervention.
SLPs have a role to play with children who have difficulty using language to learn. They need our help to develop the language base necessary for academic success.

Children who have language impairments do develop language. Their progress through the developmental stages at ages 2, 3, and 4 may be slower than that of typically developing children, but their vocabularies, syntax, and morphology do not remain static. Often, a casual conversation about a familiar topic with a school-aged child who has a language impairment may not reveal evidence of an impairment. The child's language difficulties seem to reveal themselves only when the child's processing system is stressed in some way. Lahey and Bloom (1994) suggested several factors that may result in such stress, among them the necessity for communicating about new information and the necessity to comprehend or produce language organized in complex ways. As the researchers described the situation, "some of the variability in a child's performance could be related to the ease with which mental models can be constructed and held in mind. Given familiar material, a child might express complex narratives; given unfamiliar material, the child may well be dysfluent and have difficulty expressing even a simple sequence of relations" (p. 360). This analysis suggests that the focus of intervention with school-aged children needs to be more directed toward a child's ability to use language to learn than toward language learning itself. Clinicians must analyze the ways in which a child's ability to use language in the classroom is stressed and help the child and the teacher to reduce the processing load while the child learns to use language in new and more complex ways. The intervention activities and the sample lesson plans and goals in this book are designed especially to help speech-language pathologists who may be unfamiliar with this approach to language.

Does this sort of clinical practice make a difference for children?

> We have used the approaches described in this book in real-world practice with real children for several years. Our data show that children can learn these language skills and that this knowledge has an impact on their academic success.

We have been working for the past 5 years to refine the assessment tools in this manual, and that refinement has come from asking questions about children we encountered in the schools where we worked and from listening to the questions teachers asked about what children with language impairments could do in the classroom. We have used these assessment tools to help us plan intervention and document progress resulting from that intervention. Having tested more than 300 children, we developed criterion-based scoring for use in deciding which children needed intervention. Specific pass/fail criteria in each area are described in the individual sections of the manual.

For 3 years, we conducted intervention with the children who failed to meet criterion on the tests we gave. We kept careful data about their progress, and compared it with the progress of a similar group of children in a "traditional" clinical practice focused on oral production of linguistic forms. The intervention program we developed based on our "language for learning" assessment was conducted with children in groups of three or four and, wherever possible, used topics, themes, or materials also used in the children's classrooms. Such intervention demands close collaboration with classroom teachers, and we are grateful for the generous cooperation of the teachers who have worked with us. We have conducted training with the children outside the classroom, and on occasion we have worked with an entire class at the request of a teacher. We have also worked with children in the classroom, serving as "coaches" to help a child apply what was learned in our training sessions to what the teacher was doing in the classroom. This is the kind of intervention we describe in this book.

The results of such intervention have exceeded anything we might have expected. When we began working with the children in our longitudinal research study, none of the kindergarten children and very few of the first grade children who failed to meet criterion in our assessment had been diagnosed as being in need of special services. At the end of the first year of training, over 50% of the children were able to meet criterion on the assessment tests. Of those who did not meet criterion after 1 year of training, all but one had been referred by teachers for assessment and were eventually enrolled for special education services. In other words, our training program seemed to provide us with a kind of differential diagnosis.

We discovered that kindergarten and first grade children who failed to meet criterion on our assessment, and who still did not meet criterion after a year of training in these language areas, were likely to be referred by teachers for full-range assessment. These were the children likely to end up being classified as having communication impairments, learning disabilities, or both.

What happened to the children who continued to receive training after the first year? After 2 years of training, these children also showed improvements. When compared with a similar group of children in the same school system who were not receiving training, their scores on all the assessment tasks were significantly higher. More important, their scores on a school-administered achievement test were also significantly higher.

These results seemed to us particularly significant, given that the children with whom we were working in that second year were all receiving special education services of some kind. They were the children in the caseloads of the speech-language pathologist, the learning disabilities teacher, the special education teacher, or the reading specialist. They were the children who performed in the lowest range on every academic measure tested on school achievement tests. We did not "cure" their academic difficulties. What we found, however, was that children receiving training had reading scores in the 35th percentile, while children receiving "traditional" services scored in the 20th percentile.

We discovered that even children whose academic performance is traditionally low (language impaired, learning disabled, mildly mentally handicapped) showed improvement in phonological awareness, narrative, and advanced literacy skills after 2 years of training and this improvement was also reflected in their academic performance.

We view this as a hopeful sign. Such effects suggest that what speech-language pathologists do can make a real difference for the children we serve. That is, in reality, what motivated this book.

PART I
Phonological Awareness

CHAPTER

1

Introduction to Phonological Awareness Skills

> Phonological awareness is an awareness of the individual sounds in *spoken* (not written) words that is revealed by such abilities as rhyming, isolating initial consonants of spoken words, and counting the number

Why should SLPs assess and train phonological awareness?

Speech-language pathologists in the schools have a responsibility to help children with language impairments achieve academic success. There is a large body of research indicating that a child's awareness of individual sounds in spoken words is an important precursor for early word recognition (Catts, 1989; Fletcher et al., 1994; Hatcher, Hulme, & Ellis, 1994; Stahl & Murray, 1994). The work by Stahl and Murray (1994) presents perhaps the most complete investigation of the phonological awareness/reading relationship. These researchers studied the ability of 113 kindergartners and first graders on a set of phonological awareness tasks and then compared the results to data on the children's early literacy skills. They conducted powerful statistical analyses of the data, and discovered two skills that might be thought of as foundations for reading. The first is the ability to recognize and name the letters of the alphabet, which is not, strictly speaking, a phonological awareness ability. The second, which is a phonological awareness ability, is the ability to isolate beginning and ending sounds in words. The researchers found that children in their study who could read beyond the preprimer level could also isolate beginning and ending sounds in words. They go on to say that they see phonological awareness as developing through the early grades of school as children gain greater sophistication in manipulating sounds in spoken words. The awareness that a word such as *sun* can be broken into /s/ and *un* leads to awareness that the *un* segment can be further broken up and that the *bl* in *blue* can be further broken into /b/ and /l/.

The results of this research are complemented by another line of research conducted by Bradley and Bryant (1983, 1985), addressing a sound awareness ability that seems to precede sound isolation. These researchers have shown that the ability to detect and remember rhymes is a crucial prereading ability. The reasoning suggests that attention to rhyme focuses children on sounds of words—particularly on sound at a subsyllabic level. A child who can say that *fat* and *cat* sound alike is demonstrating the ability to attend to the words' ending segments without regard to the beginning sounds.

What are the classroom implications of working with phonological awareness?

Research with kindergarten and first grade children suggests:
- First children develop a sense of rhyming through the ability to:
  - Recite familiar rhymes
  - Detect rhyme
  - Make up rhymes
- Then children develop segmentation and blending, demonstrating:
  - Attention to beginning sounds
  - Attention to ending sounds
  - Blending isolated sounds to make words
  - Phoneme addition, deletion, or movement

A brief survey of primary grade language arts curriculum materials in any elementary school will show that the ability to detect rhyme and to segment words into individual sounds is presupposed by most early reading curricula. These are abilities that many children with language impairment lack. If they are to gain access to the world of literacy, they must be helped to develop the language foundation they need. Research also shows that children can be helped to develop phonological awareness and that such development does have an impact on children's word recognition and spelling abilities (Blachman, 1991, 1994).

In the rest of this section, we will present:

- Assessment instruments to use when assessing children's ability to detect rhyme and to isolate, segment, and blend individual sounds in words.

- Information about setting criteria when using these instruments to decide if an individual child needs training in phonological awareness.
- Examples of goals and objectives useful when writing about phonological awareness on a child's individual education plan (IEP).
- Examples of lesson plans for activities designed to teach children phonological awareness.

CHAPTER

2

Assessment of Phonological Awareness Skills

As with the other abilities discussed in this book, the assessment of phonological awareness should be undertaken to determine the nature of a child's language disability rather than to determine if a language disability exists. We should be able to look at each aspect of phonological awareness to determine a child's skills at various stages along the developmental continuum.

Levels of phonological awareness
- Syllabification: most children by age 5 are able to segment words into syllables
- Rhyming: (a) remembering familiar rhymes, (b) picking out words that don't rhyme with a target word, (c) making up rhymes
- Attention to individual phonemes: isolating beginning and ending sounds of words and blending isolated sounds to make words
- Ability to add, delete, or move phonemes and regenerate the resulting word.

What should be assessed?

When planning a phonological awareness assessment, the goal is to demonstrate not only what the child cannot do but also what the child can do successfully. It is important, therefore, to have a task, or series of tasks that tap into the skills previously outlined. Therefore, in this book we include phonological awareness tasks that assess:

- Syllabification
- Rhyming
- Blending
- Sound isolation
- Segmentation
- Deletion

We choose to begin the assessment based on the child's grade level. In general, we begin with syllabification and rhyming when testing kindergarten children. We begin with blending with first and second grade children.

We have found it best to assess the kindergarten children toward the end of their first semester in kindergarten. By that time they are more acclimated to the school environment and therefore more willing to participate in the activities. Also, by the end of that first semester, the children will have benefited from the instruction in rhyming and syllabification provided by the classroom teacher.

Syllabification Task

The syllable seems to be a natural construct for children. Even a 4-year-old child who is asked to "tell me a little bit of the word *elephant*" will tell you a syllable. Of course, the child does not know the word "syllable" and it is not necessary to know the word to do this task successfully.

Materials

- You will need 6 manipulatives of any kind (i.e., small blocks, poker chips).
- You will need a list of words to use as trial items and a second list to be used as target words. The words should represent one-, two-, and three-syllable words. Appendix 2A at the end of this chapter includes a score sheet with the words that we use.

Instructions

- Place the manipulatives in a row (from left to right) in front of the child.
- Say: "We are going to break words into small pieces. Every time we hear a piece of a word, we are going to move a block. Watch while I do some."
- Say the trial word slowly, but without emphasizing each syllable. Say the trial word again, emphasizing each syllable as you move a block for each syllable. Say "See—has—pieces."

Trial Items:
    Elephant (3 syllables)
    Telephone (3 syllables)
    Hat (1 syllable)
    Pencil (2 syllables)
- Say, "Now you get to do some. Ready?" Pronounce each word clearly but at a normal rate without emphasizing the syllables. If necessary, remind the child to say the word as he or she moves the blocks. Be sure to put the blocks back in the original row before each item is presented.

Recording Responses

- Record the number of syllables the child indicated for each word. The correct response is given in parenthesis following the word on the score form. Add up the total number of correct responses.

Interpreting the Results

- We have found that it is not unusual for kindergarten children to respond correctly to four out of the five items. They most frequently miss the single-syllable word. Therefore, if a child does not get 4 out of 5 words correct, there is reason for concern.
- It should be clear when a child does not have syllable awareness. Some children just move the blocks around and some children just count the blocks.
- Note that a child must have one-to-one correspondence to understand the directions for the task.

Kindergarten Rhyming Task

Rhyming is an important foundation for becoming aware of phonemes. Rhyming leads to the ability to isolate beginning sounds. Awareness of beginning sounds is an aid in word recognition.

Rhyming is another skill that develops early in children who are exposed to it through rhyming books or games. Rhyming provides a foundation for other phonological awareness skills. A child who can detect rhyme is able to focus on the sounds rather than the meaning of words, and this shift to metalinguistic awareness is critical for early reading instruction.

Many children entering kindergarten can detect rhymes, especially if the child has had experience with rhyming. However, we have found that children from the culture of poverty often lack this experience and need a full semester in kindergarten before they can provide a true indication of their rhyming skills.

The type of task used to assess rhyming abilities is important. Many teachers begin by asking a child to tell a word that rhymes with some other word (i.e., "What rhymes with cat?"). This ability (to make up rhymes) is the rhyming skill children develop last. An easier task to determine if children understand about rhyme is a rhyme-detection task in which the child is asked to choose which word of three presented does not rhyme or "sound like" the others. This task is appropriate for children after the first semester in kindergarten. This task is also appropriate for first grade children who are having difficulty learning to read.

Materials

The pictures and the score sheet that we have used for this task are in Appendix 2B at the end of this chapter. The score sheet is arranged in three sections, which facilitate interpretation of a child's responses.

Instructions

- Say, "Some words sound alike. Cat and hat sound alike, sun and run sound alike. But cat and sun don't sound alike. Listen carefully and tell me if these two words sound alike: pat—sat. Yes, pat and sat do sound alike. Now listen again, and tell me if these two words sound alike: goat—school. No, goat and school don't sound alike." If the child does not respond appropriately, give more examples of words that sound alike and words that do not sound alike.
- Say, "Now we're going to do something else with words that sound alike. I'm going to show you three pictures, and when I name the pictures, you will hear two words that sound alike and one that doesn't belong. Let's try one."
- Trial 1: Show pictures of bell, fire, tire. Point to each picture as you name it. Give the words slowly. Ask the child to point to the one that **does not** belong.
- *Note:* if on the trial items or first item of the task the child chooses the two that rhyme, change your directions to instruct the child to point to the two that sound alike. However, you must be careful then in marking on the score sheet to circle the item that the child did **not** point to.
- Trial 2: Show the pictures of chair, bear, door. Point to each picture as you name it. Ask the child to point to the one that **does not** belong.

Note: If the child misses either trial item, repeat each with more instruction and reinforcement. It is imperative that you be sure that the child understands the task. You may repeat the trial items as many times as necessary. If the child does not seem to understand the task, even though you have made every attempt to ensure understanding, it is recommended that at least the first two sections be given. It is possible that the child will accomplish the task with further exposure. But if not, you may infer from the responses on Group 2 that the child only categorizes words by meaning.

- Proceed to item 1. Be sure to point to each picture and say the name clearly but without emphasizing the rhyme. You may repeat an entire item if you feel the child did not hear or was not attending.

Recording Responses

- On the response sheet, circle the item chosen by the child. The correct answer is printed in **bold**.
- Total the number correct for each group and for the total task.

Interpreting the Results

- As with the other assessment activities in this book, you will want to establish your own cutoff score for this task. We found that children who could not score at least 11 on this 15-point task did not demonstrate sufficient rhyming skills.
- Based on which group of words gives a child the most difficulty, we can formulate a hypothesis about the strategy that the child is using in the task. This knowledge can then be used during intervention.
- In Group 1, the odd word does not have any sound or meaning relationship with the words that rhyme (cake—lake—bat). If the child demonstrates difficulty on this section, she or he is basically guessing.
- In Group 2, the odd word has some meaning connection with one of the words that rhymes, but has no sound connection. So in Group 2, item 1 (cat—hat—mouse), if the child selects hat as the word that does not belong, the child's strategy is to pair the words semantically (cat—mouse are animals).
- In Group 3, the words all have the same middle vowel sound, so the child must attend to the final sound to determine the rhyme (man—bat—fan). Incorrect responses on this group of words indicate that the child does not pay attention to the end of the word and the answers are basically random guesses.

Assessing Advanced Phonological Awareness Skills

> **Phonological Awareness**—attending to individual sounds in spoken words, as seen in the behaviors:
>
> *Blending*—putting sounds together to make a word
>
> *Segmentation*—breaking the word apart into its individual sounds
>
> *Isolation*—identifying the individual sounds in a word (first/last)
>
> *Deletion*—removing a sound from a word

During the research process for this book, we searched the literature for an assessment tool that would evaluate all the phonological awareness processes shown to be important to a child's reading success. We felt that it was important to have a tool that would tell us both what a child could do and what the child could not do. Only with this information could we hope to plan an appropriate intervention program. We settled on the procedure described by Stahl and Murray (1994). This procedure provides the opportunity to assess a child's skills along the developmental continuum from sound blending to sound deletion. It also assesses a child's skills in each area with single sounds and blends (clusters). The tool is, therefore, suitable for first and second grade children and also for third grade children and older who are having reading difficulties.

Complete Test of Phonological Awareness

Materials

This is strictly an auditory task, as phonological awareness assesses a child's ability to understand and manipulate the sounds of words. No visual stimuli are presented.

Instructions

- The score sheet and instructions for the Complete Test of Phonemic Awareness, based on Stahl and Murray (1994), are in Appendix 2C at the end of this chapter.
- The test is made up of four sections: Blending, Isolation, Segmentation, Deletion. The instructions for each section are given in Appendix 2C at the end of this chapter. It is vital that the instructions be stated clearly and that many demonstration/trial items be presented. Each section includes trial items. If a child cannot do the task with the support provided during the trial items, he or she will have considerable difficulty on the test items. Therefore, it is imperative that the examiner makes use of the trial items to be sure a child understands the expectations.
- In each section, the items presented in the first grouping require the manipulation of the singleton. If the child cannot successfully answer 4/5 of these first items, it is appropriate to discontinue that section of the test, because the child will not be successful with the manipulation of the blends. *Example*: Section I: Blending, Part 1 Vowel-coda: If the child cannot blend these words (i.e., bad, net, etc.), you should discontinue Section I Blending and go on to Section II Isolation.
- When presenting the test items, it is crucial to present the items clearly without emphasizing the aspect that is being assessed. When presenting the Blending items, be sure to give enough pause time between the phonemes to make a clear distinction, but not such a long pause that it puts a strain on the child's working memory.
- In administering the Segmentation section, we have sometimes found it helpful to demonstrate the separation of the phonemes by using a hand

signal to further mark or emphasize the separation of the sounds. It is not necessary that a child respond with accompanying hand signals, but some do.

Recording Responses

- Mark each item as correct (+) or incorrect (−).
- Total the number of correct responses for each section and total the number of correct responses for the entire test.

Interpreting the Results

- The Compete Test of Phonemic Awareness is a criterion-referenced test and as such will need the establishment of local criteria, as discussed in the Introduction to this book.
- In the course of developing these tools, we administered the Complete Test of Phonemic Awareness to some 400 children. We found that, in general, the first grade children who demonstrated difficulty with phonological awareness scored below 35 out of the 70 points. In general, the second grade children who demonstrated difficulty with phonological awareness scored fewer than 50 to 55 out of the 70 points. It is important to remember, however, that these were children in low-income, rural community schools. It is likely that children in a different part of the country or different economic environment will have very different scores. If you prefer a more functionally based criterion, the research literature suggests that one criterion for providing intervention should be the ability to isolate beginning and ending sounds in words. As Stahl and Murray (1994) put it, "The ability to isolate a phoneme from either the beginning or the end of a word . . . seems to be crucial to reading, because nearly all children who could not adequately perform this task also had not achieved a preprimer instructional level" (p. 231). A child who cannot demonstrate this phonological awareness ability is unlikely to be able to read beyond the preprimer level. The inability to separate blends when segmenting words appeared to be a characteristic of children who were reading at a first-grade level.
- We know that phonological awareness skills are developmental in nature. As a rule, we found that first grade children could not do the deletion task, but many second graders could do it (especially by the end of the year). In general, we also found that first grade children tested in the fall of the school year were better at identifying the beginning sound in a word and had difficulty identifying the last sound in a word.
- If a kindergarten child with language impairment has difficulty with the rhyming task, it is recommended that part of the child's language intervention program be directed toward rhyming.
- If a first grade child cannot isolate the beginning sound in CVC words, it is recommended that the rhyming task be administered to determine if the child has rhyming ability.

- In general, keeping the developmental sequence in mind, it is recommended that intervention begin at the point in phonological awareness that the child is demonstrating difficulties. The next section provides goals, objectives, and sample lesson plans for the various levels of phonological awareness.

How should phonological awareness be discussed at the IEP conference?

- *Phonics* is the association of the alphabetic letter and the sound that the letter represents in words. *Phonological awareness* is the precursor to phonics.
- A child who does not understand that words are made up of individual sounds and cannot identify or manipulate those sounds is going to have a great deal of difficulty decoding (sounding out) unfamiliar words.
- The more cognitive energy a child has to expend to figure out the words, the less cognitive space the student has for understanding/comprehending what he or she is reading. This is called the processing load. When phonological awareness becomes automatic, a child can sound out words faster (more automatically) and thus can concentrate more on the meaning of what he or she is reading.
- Phonological awareness is also a key element in leaning to spell and figuring out how to spell unfamiliar words.

Summary

Phonological awareness provides the basis for reading instruction. Generally, the reading curriculum makes assumptions about children's phonological awareness abilities. Many children with language impairment do not have command of the earliest phonological awareness skills. This will set them behind their classroom peers in one more area of learning. By identifying what phonological awareness skills a child has and what skills he or she does not have, we can build an effective intervention plan that will have profound impact on the child's future academic success.

APPENDIX 2A

Syllabification Task

Name _____ School _____

Grade _____ Date _____

Directions: You will need 6 manipulatives (small blocks, poker chips). Say to the child: "We are going to break words into small pieces, and every time we hear a piece of a word, we are going to move a block. Watch while I do some."Say the trial word slowly, but without emphasizing each syllable; say the word again, emphasizing each syllable, and as you say the syllable, move a block.

   Trial items:

   Elephant (3)

   Telephone (3)

   Hat (1)

   Pencil (2)

"Now you get to do some. Ready?" Pronounce each word clearly, but at a normal rate without emphasizing the syllables.

Recording Responses: Record the number of syllables the child indicated for each word. The correct response is given in parenthesis. Add up the total number of correct responses.

1. Basketball   (3) _____

2. Monday   (2) _____

3. Paper   (2) _____

4. Dog   (1) _____

5. Principal   (3) _____

              Total _____/5

APPENDIX 2B

Kindergarten Rhyming Task

Instructions: "Some words sound alike. Cat and hat sound alike, sun and run sound alike. But cat and sun don't sound alike. Listen carefully and tell me if these two words sound alike: pat—sat. Yes, pat and sat do sound alike. Now listen again, and tell me if these two words sound alike: goat—school. No goat and school don't sound alike." If the child does not respond appropriately, give more examples of words that sound alike and words that do not sound alike.

"Now we're going to do something else with words that sound alike. I'm going to show you three pictures, and when I name the pictures, you will hear two words that sound alike and one that doesn't belong. Let's try one."

Trial 1: Show pictures of bell, fire, tire. Point to each picture as you name it. Give the words slowly. Ask the child to point to the one that **does not** belong.

> *Note:* If on the trial items or first item of the task the child chooses the two that rhyme, change your directions so that the child is instructed to point to the two that sound alike. However, you must be careful then in marking on the score sheet to circle the item that the child did **not** point to.

Trial 2: Show the pictures of chair, bear, door. Point to each picture as you name it. Ask the child to point to the one that **does not** belong.

> *Note:* If the child misses either trial item, repeat each with more instruction and reinforcement. It is imperative that you are sure that the child understands the task. You may repeat the trial items as many times as necessary. If the child does not seem to understand the task, even though you have made every attempt to ensure the child's understanding, it is recommended that at least the first two sections be given. It is possible that the child will accomplish the task with further exposure. But if not, you may infer from the responses on Group 2 that the child only categorizes words by meaning.

Proceed to item 1: Be sure to point to each picture and say the name clearly but without emphasizing the rhyme. You may repeat an entire item, if you feel the child did not hear or was not attending.

Kindergarten Rhyming Task

Score Sheet

Name _____ School _____

Grade _____ Date _____ Total _____/15

Recording responses: Circle the item the child chooses as "not belonging". The correct answers are printed in bold on the response sheet. Total the number correct in each grouping and the total number correct.

Trial 1	**bell**	fire	tire
Trial 2	chair	bear	**door**

Group 1: Words with no sound or meaning connection

1.	cake	lake	**bat**
2.	pan	fan	**kite**
3.	bees	**pig**	cheese
4.	jeep	**ball**	sheep
5.	bat	**gate**	cat

_____/5

Group 2: Words with no sound connection, but some meaning connection.

1.	cat	hat	**mouse**
2.	shell	**ring**	bell
3.	**foot**	2	shoe
4.	knee	tree	**bird**
5.	**truck**	car	star

_____/5

Group 3: Words with possible final consonant confusions

1.	man	**bat**	fan
2.	**cane**	lake	cake
3.	duck	truck	**rug**
4.	jail	**gate**	nail
5.	**wing**	ring	sink

_____/5

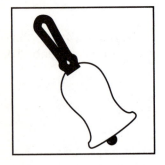
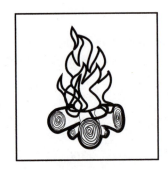
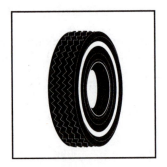

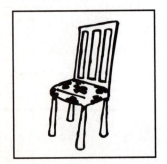
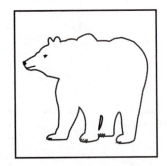
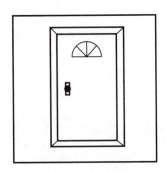

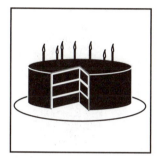
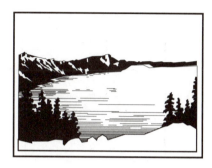
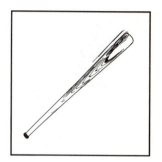

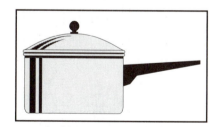
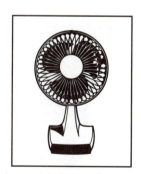
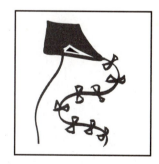

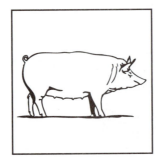

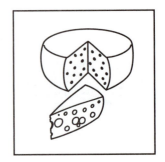

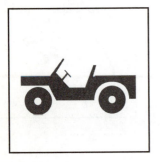

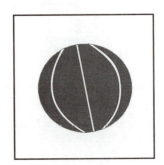

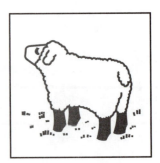

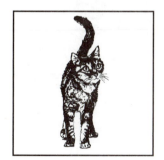 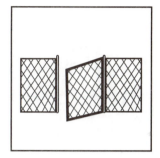 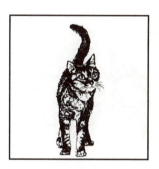

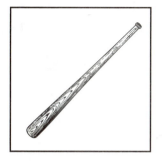  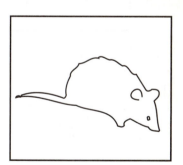

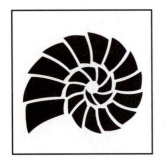 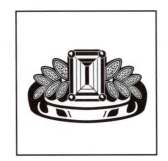 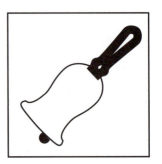

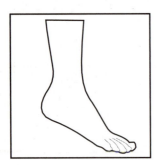 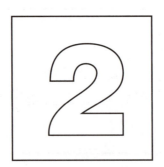 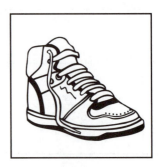

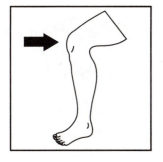

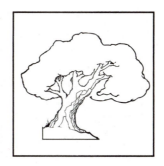

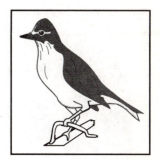

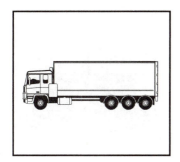

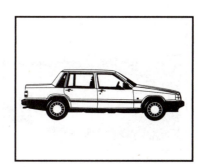

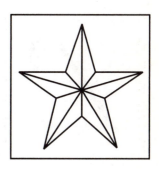

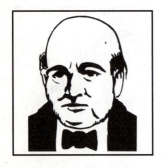 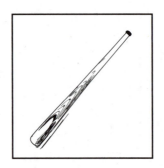 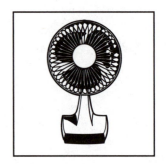

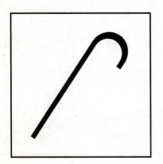 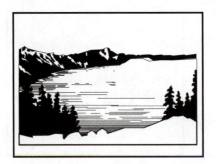 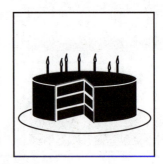

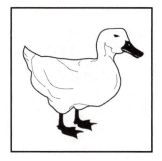

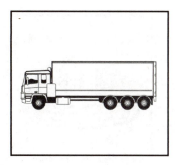

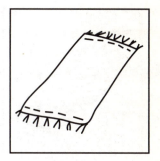

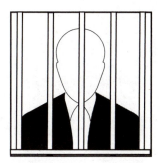

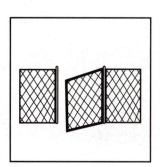

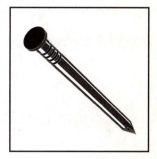

 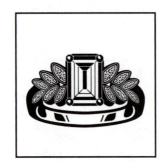 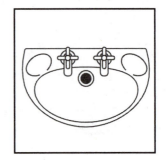

Complete Test of Phonological Awareness

Administration: For each section, give feedback only for practice words. Use additional examples if necessary. When the idea is clear, discontinue feedback and continue with test items.

I. Blending

Instructions: I'm going to say some words in a secret code, spreading out the sounds until they come out one at a time. Guess what word I'm saying. For example, if I say h-o-me, you say home. (For each item, pronounce the segments with as little additional vowel lengthening as possible).

Practice words: f-at, s-ing, s-o-me, n-o-se, s-e-n-d

II. Isolation

Instructions: This time I want you to listen for just one sound in a word. Tell me the sound you hear at the beginning of each word I say. For example, if I say food you say /f/.

Practice words: no (/n/), sheep (/ʃ/), time (/t/), hot /h/), chair (/tʃ/)

Instructions: Now I want you to listen and tell me the sound at the very end of each word I say. For example, if I say fish, you say /ʃ/. Be careful not to add any vowel onto the last sound when giving the items.

Practice words: off (/f/), mop (/p/), egg (/g/)

III. Segmentation

Instructions: Do you remember when I said the words in a secret code and you guessed what word I was saying? This time I want you to say the word in a secret code. I'll say a word, and you spread out all the sounds in the word. For example, if I say sheep you say /ʃ-i-p/.

Practice words: me (/m-i/), dish (/d-i-ʃ/), can (/k-ɑ-n/), find (/f-i-n-d/)

IV. Deletion

Instructions: I wonder if you could take a sound away from a word and make a whole new word. For example, say meat. Now say it again, but don't say /m/. (For each item, use this form: Say [word]. Now say it again but don't say [phoneme].

Practice words: cat (at), make (ache), kin (in), learn (earn)

Instructions: Now we will take the sound off the end of the word and make a whole new word. For example, say keep. Now say it again without the /p/. That's right the new word is key. Let's try some more.

Practice words: might (my), pail (pay), need (knee)

Complete Test of Phonological Awareness

Score Sheet

Name _____ School _____

Grade _____ Date _____ Total correct for the entire test _____ /70

Instructions: Score each item as correct (+) or incorrect (−). Total the number correct for each section and total the number correct for the entire test.

I. Blending

1. Vowel-coda

   b-a-d _____   t-ea-m _____

   n-e-t _____   sh-o-p _____

   s-oa-p _____

2. Cluster onset

   b-l-a-ck _____   s-p-i-n _____

   c-r-ea-m _____   p-l-a-te _____

   s-t-a-te _____

3. Cluster coda

   f-a-s-t _____   l-a-m-p _____

   p-a-r-k _____   t-o-l-d _____

   m-o-s-t _____

                                Total correct _____ /15

II. Isolation

1. Onset-rime

   foot /f/ _____   same /s/ _____

   car /k/ _____   pet /p/ _____

   seat /s/ _____

2. Cluster onset

   frame /f/ _____   spit /s/ _____

   crack /k/ _____   plane /p/ _____

   steam /s/ _____

3. Vowel-coda

   came /m/ _____   moose /s/ _____

   bat /t/ _____   bed /d/ _____

   bus /s/ _____

4. Cluster coda

   land /d/ _____   child /d/ _____

mask /k/   _____   waste /t/   _____

damp /p/   _____

Total correct   _____/20

III. Segmentation

1. Onset-rime and Vowel-coda

note /n-o-t/   _____   seed /s-i-d/   _____

game /g-e-m/   _____   fun /f-ʌ-n/   _____

sat /s-æ-t/   _____

2. Cluster onset

flake /f-l-e-k/   _____   plate /p-l-e-t/   _____

bread /b-r-ɛ-d/   _____   steam /s-t-i-m/   _____

spin /s-p-ɪ-n/   _____

3. Cluster coda

band /b-æ-n-d/   _____   bold /b-o-l-d/   _____

rank /r-æ-ɔ-k/   _____   coast /k-o-s-t/   _____

jump /dʒ-ʌ-m-p/   _____

Total correct   _____/15

IV. Deletion

1. Onset-rime

face (ace)   _____   pat (at)   _____

tin (in)   _____   page (age)   _____

same (aim)   _____

2. Cluster onset

bright (right)   _____   flag (lag)   _____

crate (rate)   _____   sleep (leap)   _____

span (pan)   _____

3. Vowel-coda

lace (lay)   _____   bead (bee)   _____

same (say)   _____   base (bay)   _____

rate (ray)   _____

4. Cluster coda

malt (mall)   _____   mold (mole)   _____

band (ban)   _____   paste (pace)   _____

bust (bus)   _____

Total correct   _____/20

Total Test   _____/70

CHAPTER

3

Intervention for Phonological Awareness Skills

Principles of Phonological Awareness Intervention

1. Acknowledge the developmental sequence that phonological awareness follows when planning intervention.

2. Use the assessment results to determine where to begin intervention.

3. Mediate for students to give them a purpose for developing phonological awareness.

4. It's never too late to start phonological awareness intervention.

5. Introduce concepts to teachers, administrators, and parents through a variety of practical strategies.

6. Integrate concepts into the language arts curriculum for all students at the elementary level (K–3).

Taking a Closer Look

Principle #1: Acknowledge the developmental sequence that phonological awareness follows when planning intervention.

- Develop goals and objectives that reflect the developmental nature of phonological awareness.
- Students progress through stages of development at their own pace. Regardless of age, follow the developmental sequence for developing phonological awareness.

- Explain the developmental sequence to older students in simple terms. Help them see the need to understand basic concepts such as rhyming first. Always use materials that are age-appropriate.

Principle #2: Use the assessment results to determine where to begin intervention.

- Develop goals and objectives that reflect a student's performance on meaningful measures of phonological awareness.
- Select assessment tools that diagnose what the student **can do** as well as what the student needs to learn.
- Begin training with all students, regardless of age, based on performance levels determined by assessment.

Principle #3: Mediate for students to give them a purpose for developing phonological awareness.

- The connection between developing phonological awareness and learning to read and write is not obvious to students.

- Explain the relationship once or twice in simple terms. Then begin each intervention lesson with a brief reminder that listening to sounds will help them to be good readers and writers.

- Mediation helps motivate students to learn difficult concepts, because it gives them a meaningful purpose.

- Mediation during phonological awareness training gives students opportunities to appreciate each of their accomplishments as they work toward learning to decode and spell written words.

Principle #4: It's never too late to start phonological awareness intervention.

- We have successfully used phonological awareness intervention with students from age 5 to age 12.
- We have observed selected students with mild to moderate developmental disabilities benefit from phonological awareness training.
- Research needs to be done with adolescents having reading disabilities.

Principle #5: Introduce concepts to teachers, administrators, and parents through a variety of practical strategies.

- Report on phonological awareness abilities in diagnostic reports shared at case conferences.
- Share research through in-service opportunities.
- Enlist the help of others in establishing local norms.
- Model instructional techniques for teachers and support staff.
- Make a presentation at a parent meeting.

Principle #6: Integrate concepts into the language arts curriculum for all students at the early elementary level (K–3).

- Participate in revisions of the language arts curriculum in your school district. A speech-language pathologist who understands the role phonological awareness plays in reading decoding and spelling can be a valuable asset to a language arts curriculum committee.
- Participate in textbook adoption. Help find a textbook series that acknowledges phonological awareness (phonemic awareness) as a precursor to phonics instruction.
- Advocate for early elementary teachers to have access to materials for teaching phonological awareness within the classroom setting.
- Offer to model instructional techniques for teachers, support staff, and parents. For example, show how spelling words can be used to practice various phonological awareness skills.

Goals and Objectives for Phonological Awareness

Our list of goals and objectives for phonological awareness represents critical skills that are typically targeted in this area. Both the goals and the objectives are stated using academically relevant terminology and can be measurable in a variety of ways. Consider this list to be a starting point when developing a program for an individual student. Use it to guide the IEP team through the goal-setting process as the issue of phonological awareness is addressed following a report of assessment results. Remember that each goal statement and objective should be modified to include measurable terms that fit the demands of the IEP format your school district has adopted.

Goal

To increase reading and writing readiness through developing phonological awareness.

Objectives

- To blend syllables into words.
- To segment words into syllables.
- To detect rhyme during shared book activities.
- To fill in rhyming words.
- To select words that belong together based on rhyme.
- To make up nonsense rhymes.
- To detect individual sounds.
- To blend CV, VC, and CVC sounds into words.
- To blend CCVC and CVCC sounds into words.
- To identify beginning sounds in words.
- To identify ending sounds in words.
- To identify middle sounds in words.
- To segment CV, VC, and CVC words into sounds.
- To segment CCVC and CVCC words into sounds.
- To remove beginning sounds and tell what word remains.
- To remove ending sounds and tell what word remains.

Goal

To increase reading decoding at the early elementary level by applying phonological awareness strategies.

Objectives

- To associate sounds with letters in the initial position of CV, VC, and CVC words.
- To associate sounds with letters in the initial position of CCVC and CVCC words.
- To associate sounds with letters in the final position of CV, VC, and CVC words.
- To associate sounds with letters in the final position of CCVC and CVCC words.
- To associate sounds with letters in the middle position of CVC words.
- To associate sounds with letters in the middle position of CCVC and CVCC words.

Goal

To increase spelling skills at the early elementary level by applying phonological awareness strategies.

Objectives

- To spell beginning sounds in CV, VC, and CVC words.
- To spell beginning sounds in CCVC and CVCC words.
- To spell ending sounds in CV, VC, and CVC words.
- To spell ending sounds in CCVC and CVCC words.
- To spell middle sounds in CVC words.
- To spell middle sounds in CCVC and CVCC words.

A Word About Our Lesson Plans for Phonological Awareness Intervention

Our goal in this section is to prepare clinicians to begin intervention in phonological awareness. We hope that clinicians will find this section helpful in their collaboration with special education and general education teachers. The sample lesson plans include valuable information meant to be shared with all those committed to improving the language arts skills of children with language impairment. Some clinicians may even find selected lessons appropriate to share with interested parents.

Each lesson plan includes:

- Introduction to procedures.
- Objectives for each lesson.
- Materials needed.

- Basic clinician script.
- Student script.
- Suggested cueing strategies.
- Suggested criteria for mastery for each lesson.

Taking a Closer Look

The **introduction** for each lesson includes a reminder of its clinical and educational relevance. It describes the role of the clinician, teachers, and parents in developing a particular skill. It also suggests various intervention contexts that have proved successful in our experience.

The **objectives** for each lesson are presented in simple form. They should be made measurable by the clinician or teacher through adding a context and criteria. Although some districts insist that progress be reported strictly in percentage of accuracy, others acknowledge that reporting gains in terms of the amount of support a child needs to maintain performance levels similar to those of peers is more meaningful.

Materials needed for each lesson are listed. Most are easily made or attainable at a local teacher supply or craft store. The children's books listed are currently in print and should be available at a local library, bookstore, or on-line book vendor. We are frequently asked about using intervention "kits." We do not use kits to teach phonological awareness. We use only the materials listed in our lesson plans.

A **basic clinician script** for each lesson is provided to give clinicians, teachers, and parents a general idea of what is said to our students as we proceed through each lesson. It is not meant to be "the only way" to talk with the students, but should give an indication of our approach. Remember that mediation and self-talk are powerful communication tools. Be sure that students know the purpose of each activity, with thinking strategies verbalized during demonstrations.

A **student script** for each lesson is provided to give clinicians, teachers, and parents an idea what students say or do when their responses are "on the right track." The scripts are based on our observations of students while learning specific concepts.

Suggested cueing strategies are described, because of the importance of providing scaffolding throughout the intervention process. The cues provided are taken directly from our clinical and classroom experiences with students. They vary in nature and intensity, depending on a student's response to a given learning opportunity. If students seem to rely too heavily on cues, consider the need for additional demonstration or teaching.

Suggested criteria for mastery of specific concepts are given for each lesson. We generally recommend reaching a mastery level of performance before proceeding to the next lesson. However, in special cases in which mastery learning is not a realistic expectation, criteria for moving to the next lesson may need to be set on an individual basis. Under these circumstances, frequent review of previously "learned" concepts through direct practice and mediation is the key to successful intervention.

Lesson Plans for Phonological Awareness Intervention

Teaching Syllabification

Introduction

Syllabification is the process of segmenting multisyllabic words into syllables. Understanding syllabification comes before understanding more abstract concepts such as segmentation of words into phonemes. Many preschool students demonstrate understanding of syllabification long before the term "syllable" is meaningful. School-aged children rely on syllabification strategies as they learn to decode and spell unfamiliar multisyllabic words.

Objectives

There are two basic objectives when teaching syllabification. One objective requires the student to blend multisyllabic words and the other requires the student to segment multisyllabic words. The objectives can be made measurable by stating the number of words the student must successfully blend or segment independently. We recommend using words from the classroom curriculum whenever possible to give the student an obvious classroom connection. Also, it is important to include phonological awareness objectives in the student's IEP. The objectives for syllabification fit logically under the goal areas of reading readiness, reading decoding, and spelling.

Materials

Few materials are needed to teach syllabification concepts. Multiple-syllable words can be taken from children's books, grade level texts, spelling lists, or vocabulary based on curriculum based thematic units. We have even used class lists with student names.

Clinician Role

The clinician's script must be consistent. Students with language impairment often become overwhelmed when the language used during instruction is too varied. Although a speech-language pathologist may initially diagnose the need for phonological awareness intervention, ideally the classroom teacher and parent will join in providing opportunities for instruction within the student's language arts curriculum. Collaboration is the key to increasing consistency among partners in education. Mediation when teaching syllabification can be as simple as explaining "breaking words into parts makes kids better readers."

Student Role

The student needs daily opportunities to learn about syllabification. Lessons provide opportunities for students to respond verbally and nonverbally. Blending and segmenting tasks teach the use of motor movements to help students mark syllables in words.

Suggested Cueing Strategies

Syllabification tasks can be made easier by presenting a closed set of words that are familiar and can be represented through pictures (such as farmer, chicken, and tractor). Selecting words that are tied to a classroom theme is also helpful. These two strategies focus a child's attention, reduce the chances of random guessing, and assure the clinician that the child has heard the target word before. Verbal cues include segmenting the first syllable of a word for the student or blending the first two syllables of a three-syllable word.

Suggested Criteria for Mastery

Mastery of syllabification is indicated when a student consistently and independently blends and segments familiar one-, two-, and three-syllable words. Another way to determine mastery is to ask the student to tell you a "little bit" of a multisyllabic word. For example, "Tell me a little bit of the word "cookie." The student should reply by saying the first or second syllable in isolation.

Lesson Plan: Syllabification

Objectives

    1. To segment words into syllables.

    2. To blend syllables into words.

Materials

- Books with one-, two-, and three-syllable vocabulary words.
- Word lists composed of one-, two-, and three-syllable words.
- Class lists with first and last names of classmates.

Activity

Play games with words containing one, two, and three syllables. Provide opportunities for students to blend syllables into words and segment words into syllables.

Procedures: Segmenting Task

Demonstration: Explain that words can be broken into parts, and each part can be said by itself. Give several examples such as, "The word *playground* has two parts. I can say each part by itself . . . *play—ground.*"

Mark each syllable by clapping.

- ○ **Clinician:** Say a two- or three-syllable word aloud.
- ○ **Student:** Segment the word into syllables by marking each syllable with a gross or fine motor movement such as clapping, stomping, or tapping. (For example, the word "elephant" could be marked with three consecutive claps.)

○ **Clinician:** Repeat the segmented syllables aloud to confirm the student's response. Provide cues if the student did not accurately segment the syllables. Acknowledge a correct response appropriately. Provide further opportunities for practice as needed.

Procedures: Blending Task

Demonstration: Explain how words that have been broken into parts can be put back together again. Give several examples such as, "Bas—ket—ball (clap-clap-clap), can be put together to make the word "basketball".

○ **Clinician:** Say a word aloud one syllable at a time (Ap—ple).

○ **Student:** Listen and blend the syllables into a word. Respond by saying the word aloud or pointing to a picture that represents the word.

○ **Clinician:** Repeat the word aloud to confirm the student's response. Provide cues if the student did not accurately blend the syllables. Acknowledge a correct response appropriately. Provide further opportunities for practice as needed.

Teaching Rhyming

Introduction

Rhyming is a phonological awareness skill that is commonly associated with preschool, kindergarten, and early elementary curriculum. Given repeated opportunities to hear rhyme in contexts such as nursery rhymes, most young children learn what rhyme "sounds like" before entering school. However, a growing number of children seem to lack awareness that words can "sound" alike. Perhaps they have been denied early literacy experiences. Perhaps they are "slow learners." Or maybe they have language impairment. Whatever the reason, developing awareness of rhyme and eventually thinking of rhyming words appear to be important steps along the way to becoming a reader.

Objectives

There are four basic objectives when teaching rhyming. Because learning about rhyme is developmental in nature, the objectives coincide with the developmental hierarchy. The first objective requires the student to detect rhyme, the second requires the student to fill in rhyming words, the third deals with making up nonsense rhymes, and the last asks the student to select words that "go together," based on rhyme. The objectives for rhyming fit logically under the goal area of reading readiness. Include them in a student's IEP when assessment indicates rhyming skills are needed.

Materials

Books, books, and more books! The most challenging and, we think, the most fun, part of teaching rhyming is finding children's books with simple rhyming patterns. Some of our favorites include:

Up Went the Goat and *The Gum on the Drum*, by B. Gregorich (both published in 1992 by School Zone Publishing Company, Grand Haven, MI)

The Fat Cat Sat on the Mat, by N. Karlin (published in 1996 by HarperCollins, New York, NY)

The Snowball, by J. Armstrong (published in 1996 by Random House, New York, NY)

Collaborate by obtaining titles from teachers and the school librarian. Borrowing and sharing materials can be a backdoor way of advertising that phonological awareness is now part of the speech-language pathologist's language curriculum.

Clinician Role

Use the word "rhyme" followed by a working definition of the term. In other words the dialogue should include frequent comments such as, "Listen, *dog—log* those words *sound alike . . .* they *rhyme.*" Draw the student's attention to words that rhyme by frequent repetition of the word pairs throughout an activity. Use of prosodic devices can be an effective strategy for making rhyming words salient. We find modifying rate, using rhythm, and varying intensity particularly helpful.

Student Role

Students benefit from daily experiences with rhyme. Informal opportunities to listen to rhyme can be created within the school routine and can be as important as specific activities. Early lessons for teaching about rhyming require sustained joint attention. The student participates largely by listening to books read aloud. Eventually, laughter or a smile as rhyme is recognized independently is considered a positive response. Later lessons require students to select a picture that completes a rhyming pair or filling in a rhyming word verbally.

Suggested Cueing Strategies

Rhyming tasks are difficult to cue without giving the student the answer. We generally control the difficulty of rhyming activities through the books we choose and the nature of the rhyming pairs we target. Children's books with minimal text and clearly pictured rhyming words are easiest. Repetition is also a strategy. We may present only one or two books per week and cycle back frequently. The rhyming pairs can be selected using the hierarchy discussed in the assessment section of this manual. For example, begin with words that have no meaning-based connection and progress to words that do.

Suggested Criteria for Mastery

Mastery of rhyming is ideal before moving on to higher levels of phonological awareness. However, experience has taught us that some students with language impairment demonstrate inconsistent awareness of rhyme through second grade. We have not delayed further phonological awareness training in these cases. However, continued opportunities to master rhyming skills have been a part of training. In general, we consider rhyme mastered when a student can independently generate several words within a word family given a CVC stimulus (such as dog-jog-log-hog) or consistently selects words that "sound alike" from a closed set of three words.

Lesson Plan: Rhyming

Objectives

1. To detect rhyme.

2. To fill in rhyming words.

3. To make up nonsense rhymes given a pattern.

Materials

Simple books with pictures that support rhyming pairs.

Activity

Reading aloud.

Procedures: Detecting Rhyme

Demonstration: Read books aloud and comment on words that rhyme. Use the term *rhyme* alternately with the phrase *sound alike*.

○ **Clinician:** Read a book aloud *slowly*. Emphasize the words that rhyme through voice (prosody) and facial expression (animated).

○ **Student:** Demonstrates sustained joint attention.

○ **Clinician:** Return to selected pages. Make comments such as, "This is my favorite page because I like the way *bears* and *stairs* rhyme. They sound *alike*."

○ **Student:** Finds a favorite page and comments about the way words sound.

Procedures: Filling in Rhyming Words

Demonstration: Read a rhyming book aloud all the way through. Comment on words that *rhyme/sound alike*. Read part of a sentence then pause, leaving out the word that completes the rhyme. Fill in the rhyming word incorrectly, then correct the mistake followed by a comment such as, "That sounds better because **house** and **mouse** *rhyme*."

○ **Clinician:** Read a book aloud *slowly*. Emphasize the words that rhyme through voice (prosody) and facial expression (animated). Leave out the word that completes the rhyme. Give the student an opportunity to fill in the rhyming word.

○ **Student:** Fill in the rhyme with the correct word.

○ **Clinician:** Acknowledge a correct response appropriately. Cue an incorrect response by asking for a word that "sounds like _____, giving an either/or choice, or pointing to a picture that represents the correct response. Provide continued opportunities for practice as needed.

Procedures: Making up Nonsense Rhymes

Demonstration: Read a rhyming book aloud all the way through. Read it a second time and follow the procedures for the "filling in rhyming words" lesson plan. Extend the experience by restating the rhyming pair and immediately adding other real and nonsense words that rhyme. For example, "cat—hat . . . bat—mat—rat—lat—jat—wat—sat—zat". Encourage students to add a real word or a silly word.

- ○ **Clinician:** Read a rhyming book all the way through. State the rhyming pair. Ask the student to add a silly word or a real word that sounds like _____ and _____.

- ○ **Student:** Add at least one word that rhymes.

- ○ **Clinician:** If the student needs a cue, give an initial continuant sound (not a letter name) and wait for a response. Repeat the rhyming pair and an initial sound so all the student needs to do is add the VC pattern to complete the rhyme (cat—hat—sss).

Lesson Plan: Rhyming

Objective

To select words that go together based on rhyme.

Materials

Pictures that represent words that rhyme (rhyming cards). The pictured items should be familiar to students. Printed words should **not** be visible.

Activity

Select two pictures that represent rhyming words from an array of three pictures.

Procedures: Selecting Rhyming Words

Demonstration: Present a target word (picture) and name it aloud. Present two more words (pictures), one that rhymes with the target and one that does not. Model self-talk strategies for comparing each word to the target. State which words "go together" and the reason. For example, "**Dog—log** or **dog—gate** . . . **dog—log** go together because they _sound alike_, they _rhyme_.

- ○ **Clinician:** Present a target picture and name it aloud. Present two more pictures, one that rhymes and a foil. Ask the student to find the one that goes with (**target**).

- ○ **Student:** Select a picture by pointing and preferably naming it aloud.

- ○ **Clinician:** Confirm a correct response appropriately. Ask the student to explain why the pictures the child selected "go together."

- ○ **Student:** "They sound alike . . . they rhyme."

- ○ **Clinician:** Cue by saying, "The words _____ and _____ go together because they _____."
- ○ **Student:** Rhyme!

Teaching Detection of Phonemes and Phoneme Blending

Introduction

Students need to learn that words are made up of individual sounds. Detecting isolated phonemes and phoneme blending is the first step. Intervention involves auditory tasks in which letter shapes and letter names are not taught. The clinician and the student communicate during activities without reference to either. Activities involve listening and manipulating sounds from the English language. Later instruction in reading decoding and spelling teaches students to match specific sounds with letters and letter patterns.

Students with limited phonological awareness benefit from listening for isolated phonemes before hearing strings of phonemes as in blending tasks. Begin activities using continuant sounds. Verbal presentation of these sounds can be sustained by the clinician and, thus, are relatively easier to detect than other sounds. With various amounts of practice, students move from successfully detecting isolated phonemes to detecting strings of phonemes and blending them into CV, VC, and CVC words.

Objectives

There are four basic objectives when teaching phoneme detection and phoneme blending. Each corresponds with a developmental step in phonological awareness.

The first objective requires the student to detect individual sounds. The next three involve blending two, three, and four sounds into monosyllabic words. Objectives for teaching phoneme detection and blending fit logically under the goal area of reading readiness. Include them in a student's IEP when assessment indicates difficulty with blending phonemes into monosyllabic words.

Materials

Some materials can be purchased, but most can be made with the help of parent volunteers. Purchased materials might include small blocks or tokens, word family cards, and children's book sets based on word families. Items are readily available through teacher's supply stores, educational merchandise catalogs, or bookstores. Simple visual aids for blending sounds into words (referred to as "say-it-move-it" boards) can quickly be mapped out on tag board with stencils or on heavy paper using basic computer graphics. (An example of a "Say-It-Move-It" board is included in Appendix 3A at the end of this chapter.)

Clinician Role

Do not talk about letter names or printed graphemes during training activities at this level of intervention. Clinical experience has taught us that students with limited phonological awareness often confuse letter names, letter shapes, and letter sounds. Although some children seem to have memorized bits and pieces of information, this appears void of any true understanding. At this stage of training, the clinician's script needs to focus the student exclusively on what the child hears. The clinician produces each consonant phoneme one time and minimizes attachment of vowels. For example, the word "bat" is presented /b/—/ae/—/t/ instead of "buuu—ae—tuuuu."

Student Role

Auditory attention and concentration will influence a student's response. During a phoneme-detection activity, the student listens to a single phoneme or a series of random phonemes presented one at a time. The student detects the individual sounds by reporting the number of sounds heard. During a phoneme blending activity, the student listens to a series of two, three, or four phonemes presented one at a time. The student blends the sounds into a real word and states it aloud.

Suggested Cueing Strategies

Visual cues and "either/or" choices are used to support students during phoneme-detection and phoneme-blending activities. During phoneme detection activities the student is cued by saying, "Listen, /f/—/m/ is either one sound or two sounds." In addition, blocks or tokens can be moved as the clinician says each sound. This "say-it-move-it" strategy provides an opportunity to determine the number of sounds heard by visually counting blocks.

The "say-it-move-it" strategy can also be helpful during phoneme blending activities. It gives the student a concrete visual representation of the number of sounds to be blended. This strategy, in combination with giving the student a closed set of words (pictures) to choose from, is particularly helpful when students have no response or are guessing words at random.

Suggested Criteria for Mastery

Mastery of phoneme detection and blending is an important step in phonological awareness intervention. It demonstrates an initial understanding that words comprise individual sounds. We consider phoneme detection and blending to be mastered when students successfully listen to CVC, CCVC, and CVCC combinations presented one sound at a time and consistently blend them to make words. Ideally, a student should not use visual supports. However, we have allowed students with significant attention and/or working memory issues to rely on the visual cues outlined earlier.

Lesson Plan: Phoneme Detection and Blending

Objectives

    1. To detect individual sounds.

    2. To blend CV and VC combinations into words.

3. To blend CVC combinations into words.

4. To blend CCVC and CVCC combinations into words.

Materials

Word lists, say-it-move-it boards, blocks or tokens, word family cards (pictures, not print), children's book sets based on word families,

Activity

With a structured format, the clinician provides opportunities for students to listen and detect individual sounds or blend combinations of sounds into words. The sources for words used in blending activities include words from classroom spelling lists or thematic units, word family cards that picture familiar items, or vocabulary from children's books.

Procedures: Phoneme Detection Task

Demonstration: The clinician models strategies for listening and counting individual sounds. A variety of single phonemes and series of up to three random phonemes are presented by tape recorder. The clinician holds up fingers or moves blocks as each sound is presented, then counts fingers or blocks and states the number of sounds heard. Students are encouraged to count along with the clinician.

- ○ **Clinician:** Beginning with continuant sounds, produce one phoneme slowly. Ask students, "How many sounds did you hear?" Provide visual support cues as outlined in **Teaching: Phoneme Detection and Phoneme Blending** as needed.

- ○ **Student:** Count the phoneme heard and state, "I heard one sound."

- ○ **Clinician:** Repeat the procedures, using a variety of consonant sounds and vowels (no diphthongs). Try not to attach a schwa vowel to a stop consonant. Next use strings of two and three random phonemes. Ask students, "How many sounds did you hear?" Provide visual support cues as outlined in **Teaching: Phoneme Detection and Phoneme Blending** as needed.

- ○ **Student:** Count the phonemes heard and state, "I heard ____ sounds."

Procedures: Phoneme Blending Task

Demonstration: The clinician models strategies for listening and blending individual sounds into words. Begin with CV and VC words and work up to CCVC and CVCC words. Present words one sound at a time using a tape recorder. Demonstrate active listening by using self-talk (repeat the sounds slowly to yourself) or use the say-it-move-it strategy to assist students in blending sounds into words. State the word aloud. Encourage students to participate.

- ○ **Clinician:** Begin with words that have continuant sounds (me, fall, sunny). Produce a word slowly, one sound at a time. Ask students, "What word did you hear?" Provide visual support cues as outlined in **Teaching: Phoneme Detection and Phoneme Blending** as needed.

○ **Student:** Blend the phonemes and state the word aloud.

○ **Clinician:** Present a variety of two-, three-, and four-sound words (toe, dog, skate). Produce a word slowly, one sound at a time, minimizing attachment of schwa vowels. Ask students, "What word did you hear?" Provide visual support cues as outlined in Teaching: Phoneme Detection and Phoneme Blending as needed.

○ **Student:** Blend the phonemes and state the word aloud.

Teaching Phoneme Isolation

Introduction

The ability to isolate phonemes in all positions of words is at the heart of learning to read and spell. Following a review of "letters and sounds," the early phonics curriculum introduces the concept of "beginning sounds." Before long, first grade students are expected to fill in, spell, and decode beginning sounds in words. Later on, the concepts of middle and ending sounds are introduced.

Some students with limited phonological awareness get enough practice labeling "beginning sounds," that they can complete basic worksheets with little assistance. However, the teacher usually notes minimal carryover of the skill to decoding and spelling activities. In fact, our experiences with assessment have found that many students capable of isolating beginning sounds in a structured task cannot blend sounds into words or meaningfully use their knowledge of beginning sounds. They have apparently memorized the task in one context and have no functional understanding of the role sounds play in words.

Objectives

There are three basic objectives when teaching phoneme isolation: to identify sounds in the initial position of words, the final position of words, and lastly the medial position of words. Three separate objectives are necessary, because students do not acquire these skills all at once. The objectives for teaching phoneme isolation fit logically under the goal area of reading readiness. Include one, two, or all three of them in a student's IEP when assessment indicates difficulty with isolating phonemes.

Materials

Some materials can be purchased, but most can be made with the help of parent volunteers. Purchased materials might include small blocks or tokens, word family cards, and children's book sets based on word families. Items are readily available through teacher's supply stores, educational merchandise catalogs, or bookstores. Simple visual aids for phoneme isolation (referred to as "say-it-move-it" boards) can quickly be mapped out on tag board with stencils or on heavy paper using basic computer graphics.

Clinician Role

Letter names and letter shapes are not discussed during phoneme isolation activities. The clinician's dialogue refers only to what the student hears. The clinician's production of each consonant phoneme should be clear and minimize attachment of vowels as much as possible. Some language arts curricula refer to a phoneme as a *beginning, middle, or ending* sound; others use the terms *first, middle, and last.* Clinicians should always use terminology consistent with the district language arts curriculum during phonological awareness intervention to support carryover of skills.

Student Role

Students often respond with letter names during phoneme isolation activities.

In fact, the tendency to use letter names when asked, "What *sound* do you hear?" is quite typical. After all, parents and most early childhood programs focus on letter names long before they teach the *sounds* letters represent. Students must be required to respond during phonological awareness training by producing the *sound* they heard.

Suggested Cueing Strategies

Visual support and "either/or" choices are used to assist students during phoneme isolation activities. The "say-it-move-it" strategy is helpful because the blocks or tokens are moved as the clinician says each sound. It gives the student a concrete visual representation of the particular position of each sound. A different colored block/token can be used to highlight the position of the sound being isolated. Giving the student an either/or choice is also an effective strategy, particularly when students have no response or guess sounds at random.

Suggested Criteria for Mastery

Mastery of sound isolation is gradual. First, students master isolation of initial phonemes. The clinician asks the student, "What's the beginning sound in the word _____?" and the student consistently responds by producing the initial phoneme in isolation. Next, students master isolation of final phonemes. The clinician asks, "What's the ending sound in the word _____?" and the student consistently responds by producing the final phoneme in isolation. Finally, the student masters isolation of medial phonemes. The clinician asks, "What's the middle sound in the word _____?" and the student consistently responds by producing the medial phoneme in isolation.

Our experience teaching phoneme isolation indicates that students typically reach a high level of accuracy isolating initial phonemes before the ability to isolate final and medial phonemes emerges. In fact, some students continue to struggle with isolating sounds in the final and medial positions of words, unless the word is *segmented* (produced one sound at a time) by the clinician using a say-it-move-it board. Frequently, we have introduced the next skill (segmenting words into sounds) while continuing to provide opportunities to isolate final and medial sounds.

Lesson Plan: Phoneme Isolation

Objectives:

1. To identify beginning sounds in CV, VC, CVC, CCVC, and CVCC words.
2. To identify ending sounds in CV, VC, CVC, CCVC, and CVCC words.
3. To identify middle sounds in CVC, CCVC, and CVCC words.

Materials

Word lists, say-it-move-it boards, blocks or tokens, word family cards (pictures, not print), children's book sets based on word families,

Activity

The clinician provides opportunities for students to listen to words and isolate phonemes in the initial, final, or medial position in a structured format. The sources for words used in phoneme isolation activities include words from classroom spelling lists or thematic units, word family cards that picture familiar items, or vocabulary from children's books.

Procedures: Phoneme Isolation Task

Demonstration: First, explain that all words have a beginning sound and an ending sound. Next, explain that most words have at least one middle sound. Then remind students that the reason they practice listening and telling about sounds in words is to help them with reading.

Introduce the source for the words being used in the lesson. If a book is the source, cover the print and read it aloud from a separate script. Next, explain the objective of the lesson. (Indicate whether to listen for the beginning, middle, or ending sound.) Choose words with two or three sounds. Words with continuant sounds are easiest (saw, shoe, mom, fall).

Choose a CVC word from the source being used in the lesson. Say it aloud. Then say it one sound at a time. Using the say-it-move-it board, slide a block to represent each sound as you say it aloud. Point to the first block and say, "The beginning sound in the word 'fan' is /f/." Provide as many demonstrations as needed to familiarize students with the task.

- ○ **Clinician:** Say a word aloud one sound at a time. Use the say-it-move-it board to move a block for each sound. Ask the students, "What word did you hear?"
- ○ **Student:** Blend the sounds into a word and say the word aloud.

- ○ **Clinician:** Ask the student, "What was the first sound you heard in the word _____?" If the student needs a cue, say and show the word again one sound at a time using the say-it-move-it board. Point to the position of the beginning sound on the say-it-move-it board. Prolong the sound if necessary to give it emphasis.

- ○ **Student:** State the beginning sound in the target word and say it aloud.

- ○ **Clinician:** Affirm a correct response appropriately by saying, "Right, the beginning sound in the word 'mom' is /m/." Cue an incorrect response by saying and showing the word one sound at a time and pointing to the block that goes with the beginning sound.

Note: Follow the same basic procedures for isolating ending and middle sounds in words. When isolating initial sounds in CCVC words, we treat the initial blend as two sounds. In other words, the beginning sound in the word "stop" is /s/. When isolation final sounds in CVCC words, we treat the final blend as two sounds as well. So, the final sound in the word "lamp" is /p/. We treat the /t/ in "stop" and the /m/ in "lamp" as middle sounds.

Teaching Segmentation of Words into Phonemes

Introduction

Segmenting words into phonemes is the foundation for independent decoding of unfamiliar words and using logical invented spelling. The language arts curriculum typically assumes that early elementary students have the ability to segment simple words into as many as four individual sounds. Students with reading decoding difficulties and illogical invented spelling often have limited ability to segment words into as few as two and three phonemes. It seems that, without the underlying ability to break up words into individual sounds, even a student who knows the letter names, letter sounds, and how to write the alphabet has a good chance of being described as "behind" in reading by the middle to end of first grade.

Objectives

There are three basic objectives when teaching how to segment words into phonemes. They begin with breaking up CV and VC words into phonemes, move to segmenting CVC words, and end with dividing CCVC and CVCC words into individual sounds. The objectives for teaching these skills are written in a developmental sequence and fit logically in the goal area of reading readiness. Include one or all of these objectives in a student's IEP if assessment indicates difficulty with segmenting words into phonemes.

Materials

The materials needed for teaching segmentation of words are much the same as for teaching earlier phonological awareness skills. Some materials can be purchased but most can be made with the help of parent volunteers or classroom assistants. Purchased materials might include small blocks or tokens, word family cards (pictures only), and children's book sets based on word families. These items are readily available through teacher's supply stores, educational merchandise catalogs, or bookstores. Simple visual aids for segmenting words into phonemes (referred to as "say-it-move-it" boards) can quickly be mapped out on tag board with stencils or on heavy paper using basic computer graphics.

Clinician Role

We do not use the word "segment" during instruction. We refer to segmentation as breaking words up or saying a word one sound at a time. Sound-symbol correspondence is not discussed during phonological awareness training at this stage. The clinician's dialogue refers only to the *sounds* the student says and hears. If a student responds with the name of a letter, we remind the child that we are talking about the sounds in words not the letters that spell the sounds.

Student Role

Each word must be segmented one *sound* at a time. Some students attempt to segment words by saying letter names one at a time, especially if they happen to know how a word is spelled. Another source of confusion can be classroom phonics instruction. If the student is learning how to spell sounds and at the same time participating in phonological awareness intervention, the terms "letter" and "sound" may be getting confused.

Suggested Cueing Strategies

Visual support cues are most helpful when learning to segment words into phonemes. During early instruction, the say-it-move-it strategy allows the student to physically move a block or token as a word is segmented. The say-it-move-it strategy also provides a framework for cueing. If a student segments a word too quickly and indicates that it has four sounds when it actually has three, the clinician can model how to segment the word correctly by moving a block or token to represent each sound in the word.

Suggested Criteria for Mastery

Segmenting words into phonemes is mastered when a student can consistently segment words containing up to four sounds. Ideally, the student should not need visual support such as a say-it-move-it board. However, we have had students who used tally marks or asked for blocks during post-test sessions and segmented every word correctly. In these cases, we assumed that eventually the student would not need these supports and moved on to the final level of training.

Lesson Plan: Segmentation of Words into Phonemes

Objectives

1. To segment CV and VC words into phonemes.
2. To segment CVC words into phonemes.
3. To segment CCVC and CVCC words into phonemes.

Materials

Word lists, say-it-move-it boards, blocks or tokens, word family cards (pictures, not print), children's book sets based on word families.

Activity

Within a structured format, the clinician provides opportunities for students to listen to words and segment them into individual phonemes. Simple tools are used, which makes the task hands-on and visual. The sources for words used in these activities include words from classroom spelling lists or thematic units, word family cards that picture familiar items, or vocabulary from children's books.

Procedures: Segmentation of Words into Phonemes

Demonstration: First, remind students that words are made up of sounds. Then, explain that good readers can listen to words and break them up by saying the sounds one at a time. Tell students that they will learn to break up words into sounds to help their reading.

Next, present three pictures that represent CVC words. Ask students to choose a word. Say the word slowly enough for students to hear it segmented into individual sounds.

Last, ask students to choose another word. Explain to students that a say-it-move-it board can help break up a word into sounds and place one within reach. Repeat the target word aloud. Now say it again one sound at a time. Slide a block from one end of the say-it-move-it board to a "beginning sound" position at the other end of the board as you say the initial phoneme. Slide a second block from one end of the say-it-move-it board to a "middle sound" position at the other end of the board as you say the medial phoneme. Slide a third block from one end of the say-it-move-it board to a "final sound" position at the other end of the board as you say the final phoneme.

In other words, if the student selects a picture of a "sun", say /s/ while you slide a block to an initial position space holder, /ʌ/ while you slide a block to a medial position space holder, and /n/ while you slide a block to a final position space holder. Do as many demonstrations each session as needed.

- **Clinician:** Present three pictures. Ask a student to choose a word and say it aloud. Ask the student to break up the word into sounds by saying it slowly one sound at a time. Encourage the student to use a say-it-move-it board. Remind the student to slide one block as each sound is said aloud.

- **Student:** Say the target word one sound at a time using the say-it-move-it procedure.

- **Clinician:** Ask a student to choose another word without telling the choice. Ask the student to break up the word by saying it one sound at a time using the say-it-move-it procedure. Tell the student you will guess the word by blending the sounds.

○ **Student:** Choose a word and segment it into phonemes using the say-it-move-it procedure.

○ **Clinician:** Blend the sounds and guess the word.

Teaching Phoneme Deletion

Introduction

Deleting initial or final phonemes is the final step in teaching phonological awareness. Activities beyond this level begin to teach sound symbol correspondence. We teach deletion as an extension of segmenting words into phonemes once a student has mastered that skill.

Objectives

There are four basic objectives when teaching phoneme deletion. Two of them address removal of initial phonemes and two of them address removal of final phonemes. Again, include these objectives in a student's IEP, if appropriate under the goal area of reading readiness.

Materials

The materials needed for teaching phoneme deletion are much the same as for teaching earlier phonological awareness skills. Some materials can be purchased but most can be made with the help of parent volunteers or classroom assistants. Purchased materials might include small blocks or tokens, word family cards, and children's book sets based on word families. These items are readily available through teacher supply stores, educational merchandise catalogs, or bookstores. Visual supports can quickly be mapped out on tag board with stencils or on heavy paper using basic computer graphics.

Clinician Role

We do not use the word "deletion" during instruction. We talk about "taking off" a sound from a word and telling what "new" word is left. Many students find it helpful to segment a given word (with or without a say-it-move-it board) and then remove the initial or final sound and tell what remains.

Student Role

Only one sound is removed during deletion tasks. Students tend to remove more than one sound, given CCVC and CVCC words. They also tend to attach vowels to consonants. The student should always say the target word aloud before deleting a sound. We encourage students to "think out loud" as they go through the process of phoneme deletion.

Suggested Cueing Strategies

Visual support cues are also helpful when learning to delete phonemes in the initial or final position of a word. During early instruction, the say-it-move-it strategy allows the student to physically move a block/token as a phoneme is deleted. The say-it-move-it strategy also provides a framework for cueing. Let's say a student deletes the first two sounds in a word instead of just the first sound. In this case, the say-it-move-it strategy gives the clinician an opportunity to lend visual support by first showing the student the word one sound at a time and then physically removing a block that represents just the first sound.

Suggested Criteria for Mastery

Phoneme deletion is mastered when a student can consistently delete initial and final sounds in words containing up to four sounds. Preferably, the student successfully manipulates initial and final sounds without relying on visual support. However, we have worked with some students in which criteria for mastery permitted use of the say-it-move-it strategy as long as the student used it independently.

Lesson Plan: Phoneme Deletion

Objectives

1. To remove beginning sounds in CVC words and tell what word remains.
2. To remove ending sounds in CVC words and tell what word remains.
3. To remove beginning sounds in CCVC and CVCC words and tell what word remains.
4. To remove ending sounds in CCVC and CVCC words and tell what word remains.

Materials

Word lists, say-it-move-it boards, blocks or tokens, word family cards (pictures, not print), children's book sets based on word families.

Activity

Within a structured format, the clinician provides opportunities for students to manipulate sounds in the initial and final positions of words. Simple tools are used which makes the task hands-on and visual. The sources for words used in phoneme deletion activities include words from classroom spelling lists or thematic units, word family cards that picture familiar items, or vocabulary from children's books.

Procedures: Phoneme Deletion Task

Demonstration: Explain that good readers and spellers can make "new" words by taking off beginning (or, later on, ending) sounds and blending the sounds that are left over into a word. Tell students that they will learn to take off sounds and make new words, so that learning to read and spell will be easier.

Remind students that a say-it-move-it board helps break up word into sounds, and place one within reach. Select a target word that will *remain a real word* when the initial phoneme (or later on the final phoneme) is deleted. Say the word aloud then segment it using the say-it-move-it procedure.

Physically remove the block/token from the initial position on the say-it-move-it board and repeat the initial phoneme being deleted. For example if the target word is /k/—/ae/—/t/ (cat), segment the word using the say-it-move-it procedure. Then remove the block that represents /k/ and say, "If I take off the /k/ in the word cat the leftover sounds are /ae/—/t/. . . at."

- ○ **Clinician:** Say a word that becomes a "new" word when the initial sound is removed. Ask the student to say the word, break it up into sounds, take off the beginning sound, and tell what "new" word is left over.

- ○ **Student:** Say the word, segment the word and remove the beginning sound using the say-it-move-it procedure. Tell what "new" word remains.

- ○ **Clinician:** Acknowledge a correct response appropriately. Provide additional demonstration, if necessary. Begin with words containing three phonemes and progress to words containing four phonemes.

Note: Complete this activity with deletion of ending phonemes, once mastery of initial phonemes is evident.

APPENDIX 3A

Sample Say-It-Move-It Board

The manipulatives stay in this box until the word has been given.

This is the "holding place."

The clinician can make as many squares here as necessary (up to four).

The student moves one manipulative for each sound
from the "holding place" to the square below

PART II
Narrative

CHAPTER

4

Introduction to Narrative Skills

> Narrative might well be considered the solution to a problem of general concern, namely, the problem of translating *knowing* into *telling*.

Hudson and Shapiro (1991) suggest that four kinds of knowledge are involved in a child's comprehension and production of narratives:

- *Content knowledge*—this might be called the child's world knowledge, and it includes generalized event representations (what happens at a birthday party), memories of specific events in the child's life (what happened at my sister's birthday party), memories of stories the child has heard or read, and knowledge about common types of social interactions.
- *Structural knowledge*—this is a child's knowledge about the structural components of different types of narratives. For example, what is different about the structure of an account you might give a neighbor of your own family's trip to Disney World versus the structure of a story you might write about a boy who gets lost in Disney World? In our discussion of this type of knowledge, we refer to a child's knowledge of *frameworks*, which might be thought of as generalized mental models of the structure of different types of narratives.

- *Microlinguistic knowledge*—this is, in the most general sense, a child's knowledge of the syntax and semantics of language. It includes knowledge of cohesive devices, adjustment of verb tenses, and use of pronouns and anaphoric reference, to give a few examples.
- *Contextual knowledge*—this covers a child's beliefs about the function of a narrative in a specific context. For example, is the child telling about an experience because he or she wants to share information with a group of friends, or is the child composing a story in response to a teacher's assignment?

The adequacy of a child's knowledge in each of these areas is reflected in the organization and coherence of narratives the child produces and in the ability to comprehend the most important information in narratives he or she reads or hears.

Why should SLPs assess and train a child's knowledge of narrative structure?

The research literature in the field makes it clear that children who can use narrative frameworks to structure their production of narratives produce longer, more linguistically complex narratives. Children who are able to use narrative frameworks to guide their comprehension of narratives they read or hear have better recall for information and are able to focus on what is important. (Hudson & Nelson, 1983; Lahey & Bloom, 1994; Nelson & Gruendel, 1986). This suggests that a child's ability to use a narrative framework will impact what the child does in the classroom, whether the task at hand involves reading comprehension or composing a story. Children who are unable to use structural knowledge (narrative frameworks) in common classroom situations will be at a distinct disadvantage. This is, in part, because they are likely to be overwhelmed by the processing demands of tasks such as writing a story when they are unable to support their linguistic endeavors with a narrative framework.

What are the classroom implications of training a child's ability to use narrative frameworks?

> Narrative development involves more than knowledge of narrative structure; it involves being able to hold in mind a complex model of relations among events while using language to express these relations.
> Lahey and Bloom (1994), p. 358

When we work with children who have language impairments, one of our tasks is always to try to reduce the processing demands of their classroom tasks. When a child's ability to comprehend and produce language is demanding in and of itself, whether because the child has difficulty finding the words needed to express content or because the child has difficulty constructing complex sentences to express relations between ideas, any additional processing demand is likely to overwhelm the student. One reason why so many children with language impairments may be able to produce fairly lengthy monologues when they talk and, yet, apparently are unable to produce more than two or three sentences when they are asked to write relates to the additional processing demands imposed by forming letters and spelling words. Lahey and Bloom (1994) suggested that children's ability to construct and hold in the mind mental models of the content they wish to express plays a large role in determining how demanding a specific task will be for a child. They used this idea to explain some of the variability we see in the language performance of children across time and across tasks. As Lahey and Bloom put it, "Some of the variability in a child's performance could be related to the ease with which mental models can be constructed and held in mind" (p. 360). Talking about familiar content that is supported by a familiar narrative framework allows a child to construct more complex narratives. Given unfamiliar content and an inability to access a supporting narrative framework, a child will have difficulty constructing any kind of narrative at all. Training helps to strengthen a child's knowledge of narrative structure and helps the child understand how to use this knowledge in producing and comprehending classroom-related narratives.

In the rest of this section, we present:

- Assessment procedures for eliciting and evaluating the adequacy of a child's verbalization of script frameworks, procedures for eliciting and evaluating a child's personal event narratives, and procedures for eliciting and evaluating a child's use of a story framework in a story retelling task.
- Information about setting criteria when using these assessment procedures to decide if an individual child needs training in the use of narrative frameworks.
- Examples of goals and objectives useful when writing about narrative on a child's IEP.
- Examples of lesson plans for activities designed to help children use narrative frameworks in a variety of narrative tasks.

CHAPTER

5

Assessment of Narrative Skills

> It is important that the SLP approach the task of narrative assessment with a clear sense of what information is needed to evaluate children's narrative competence.
>
> Naremore (1997), p. 21

As with any other aspect of assessment, our planning is guided by the questions that need to be answered in the assessment procedures. The following questions should guide the planning of a narrative assessment:

1. Does this child have experience with the event, so that a script might have been formed? This is a question about content knowledge. A child cannot be expected to discuss something about which he or she has no world knowledge.

2. Can the child use the script to act out (without the necessity for language) a narrative about the event? This question deals with a child's ability to use structural knowledge (script knowledge) without the added processing demands of using language.

3. Can the child compose a verbal account of the event? This looks at a child's ability to join structural knowledge and linguistic knowledge together in a single narrative event.

4. Can the child retell a well-formed story involving the event? This question addresses a child's ability to use two kinds of structural knowledge—scripts and story frameworks—together with linguistic knowledge in a single narrative event.

5. Can the child answer factual recall and inferencing questions about the story? This is about a child's ability to use structural knowledge to aid in comprehension and recall of content.

6. Can the child compose a well-formed story built on the scripted event? This question explores a child's ability to use structural and linguistic knowledge to construct and verbalize new content (Naremore, 1997, pp. 21–22).

In general these questions reflect levels of difficulty with narration. The level of difficulty is a function of the processing load or processing demands required by the task. As stated in the Introduction, the task is not to find out what the child cannot do, but to determine the circumstances (processing demands) that allow the child to do the task. Clearly, acting out a script is easier than converting the script into linguistic form as required in composing a verbal account. Also retelling a well-formed story is easier than composing a well-formed story. With these questions in mind, one can move up or down the continuum of difficulty to locate the level at which a child is successful. Or put another way, one moves up and down the continuum until the point at which the child's narrative skill "breaks down" is determined. In this manner, the appropriate level to begin intervention is found.

Assessing Scripts

Why is it important to assess script knowledge?

- It is clear that scripts are used as frameworks to describe routine events and as aids for remembering specific instances of particular events. Each new experience that a child has with a particular event enriches his or her knowledge of the script framework for that event. The framework is then used when the child is asked to read and comprehend or write about a character's experience with an event

- Using existing scripts aids in both producing and comprehending script-based narratives, because the use of the framework reduces the processing demands of a task. A script provides a child with an organizational framework for the content, and a support for recall.

How should script knowledge be assessed?

Young children learn scripts through experience. For example a 3-year-old child learns a birthday party script as a result of going to at least one birthday party. With more experiences, the child adds elaboration to the personal script. Therefore, it is necessary to determine what experiences a child has had before attempting to assess the child's ability to convert the experience into a linguistic form. Because our culture is so diverse and individual differences can be very important in script assessment, it is dangerous to assume every child of a particular age has had the same experiences and, therefore, has the same script knowledge.

How can the SLP find out about a child's scripts?

- The easiest way to determine if a child has a script is to watch the child. If she follows her classroom routine, such as storing coats and materials, taking her seat, following directions, lining up, and so on, without undue difficulty it can be assumed that the child has a classroom script.
- A brief questionnaire sent to the parent will reveal the nature of experiences that a child has had. Questions such as: How frequently does your child go to the grocery store with you? How frequently has the child been to children's birthday parties? Does your child have a bedtime routine (such as bath, tooth brushing, story, etc.) Which of the following food preparation tasks would you expect your child to know how to do: making peanut butter and jelly sandwiches? making a bowl of cereal with milk? making scrambled eggs? making pizza in the microwave? (Naremore, 1997).

Once it is determined what scripts a child has, we can decide to answer either question #2 or question #3 from the list at the beginning of this chapter. Generally, most school clinicians would probably choose to determine the answer to question #3 (Can the child compose a verbal account of the event?). Then, if necessary, back up to question #2 (Can the child use the script to act out, without the necessity for language, a narrative about the event?). However, for this discussion, we proceed through the questions in numerical order.

Can a child use the script to act out a narrative?

Materials

You will need manipulatives appropriate to the script you have chosen. If you are using a visit to the doctor script, for example, you will need a toy stethoscope, thermometer, a tongue depressor, and so on.

If you choose not to have a child actually act out a script, the same information can be gained by providing the child with a series of pictures of a person participating in the script. For example, a child in the doctor's waiting room, a child getting an examination (temperature taken, heart checked, ears examined, medicine administered, etc).

Procedure

To encourage the child to "act out" a script, we set up the scenario. Something like, "I have to go to the doctor, this afternoon. I don't know what to do when I go to the doctor. Maybe you can show me what to do and what the doctor will do. You be the doctor." We then pretend to enter the doctor's office.

If you choose not to "act out" the script, you can ask the child to arrange a picture to show what happens when you go to the doctor. This is an artificial task devoid of any context. It is helpful, therefore, to provide the child with a reason for completing this task. The clinician says, "I have a friend just your age. He is sick and has to go to the doctor. He has never been to the doctor before and is a little scared. I thought it would help him, if someone his age told him about going to the doctor. So you arrange these pictures to tell about going to the doctor and then I will show them to my friend."

Can a child compose a verbal account of an event?

What we are asking here is, can the child convert script knowledge into linguistic form? It is important that we recognize again that asking for a script is an artificial task. Generally we use the script as a basis for telling about an event or sharing an experience. We do not generally talk about a script outside of a particular experience with the scripted event. We talk, for example, about a friend's wedding not what happens when you go to a wedding.

Materials

No particular materials are necessary. It is sometimes helpful to have a general picture of the target event to provide a reason for asking for the script. We may have a picture of children entering a school building, for example, and use that as the catalyst for discussing the going to school script.

Procedure

Because discussing a script is a very decontextualized task, it is vitally important to provide an audience and a reason for the task. The clinician may say something like, "I have a friend who lives in another country, but he will be coming to America to go to school soon. He is a little afraid about going to school in America. If you tell him what happens when you go to school, I will play the tape for him."

It is very important to phrase the request "Tell what happens when . . ." It must be clear through the request that a script is called for, not a retelling of a particular event.

Demonstration

For some children it will be necessary to demonstrate the telling of a script to provide a child with an example of the type of language to be used in a script-telling task. In this case, one needs to be sure to use the linguistic form "you" and the language convention for temporal or causal relationships that denote a script telling. For example: "This weekend I was going to ride my bike, but I found I had a flat tire. When you have a flat tire you take the tire off the bike. Then you put it in a pail of water and watch for bubbles that show where the hole is. Then you put a patch on the tire to cover the hole. After the tire is fixed, you put it back on your bike and you are ready to ride."

Example Scripts

All of these scripts were gathered after determining that each child had experience with fishing.

Example 1—This is an example of a good script. Note the use of the word "you" and the use of present tense. Note also the child used both a temporal organization ("get your fishing rod . . . then you get in the boat") and a causal organization ("If you get a bite . . .").

Adult: Tell me what you do when you go fishing.

Child: Well, you get your fishing rod and your bait, and then you get in the boat. If you're going to be out very long, you probably take some water and maybe some food along. Then you get to the place where you want to anchor, and you put the bait on the hook and throw out the line and wait to see if you get a bite. If you get a bite, you pull up really fast so the fish won't get away. Then you take the fish off the hook and put it on the stringer, where you keep all the fish you catch.

Example 2—This child evidently misinterpreted the cue. In any case for some reason the student tells about one particular experience.

Adult: Tell me what you do when you go fishing.

Child: Well, I have to go with my dad, and we just get our rods and stuff and we go to the lake and get in the boat and fish. One time when we went out, it started to rain and we just stayed out there because the fish were really biting and we didn't want to leave.

Example 3—This child started with a script, but strayed into a personal narrative. This may indicate that, although the child had some knowledge of script, he could not hold it and at the same time convert it into linguistic form.

Adult: Tell me what you do when you go fishing.

Child: You get all your stuff, like your rod and your gear, and you go out to the lake and get a boat and take it out. One time when me and my brother went we seen four snakes in the water. We got out of here in a hurry, man. We didn't want to be catching snakes.

Example 4—This child demonstrated knowledge of script but did not provide much detail. It appears that this child may have word-finding difficulties that make it harder for him to attach words to the script framework.

Adult: Tell me what you do when you go fishing.

Child: Well, you get all your stuff, like, you know, your thing that you catch the fish with, and worms or crickets or stuff. Then you go out to the lake, and maybe you just stand on that wood place that goes out in the water, you know, or maybe you get a boat. And you put your worm or whatever on your hook and you just throw it in the water and wait for the fish to bite it.

Interpreting the Results

The only way to determine if a child's script telling was adequate is to compare the telling with other children from the student's classroom. Refer to the section on criterion-referenced testing in the Introduction

Transcribe the children's retelling and look for commonalties among the scripts.

There are many individual differences in experience, which can have an impact on scripts. It is not unusual for each child to display some idiosyncratic aspects of the particular script.

There are no hard-and-fast guidelines at this time to help us determine what should be in a child's script. It is known that the script should contain the word "you." If the child uses "I," he or she is giving a personal narrative rather than a script. The script should show organization and this organization should be logical either in terms of time order or causal organization. For example, you cannot put the patch on a tire until you know where the hole is.

Why might a child not do well on a script-telling task?

All cognitively normal children develop scripts. Watch a child playing a game or participating in an event and it is clear that the child has a script and is using this script knowledge to function in the event The concern here is not the presence or absence of a script, but the child's ability to verbalize the script. Verbalizing a script places demands on the linguistic system that will tax the language abilities of some children. Even with the script illustrated for them, some children will have difficulty organizing and ordering the task. (Naremore, Densmore, & Harman, 1995).

- A child with language impairment may have difficulty attaching verbal labels to elements within a script or in retrieving those verbal labels. Or the child may have the label, but because of word-finding difficulty, he cannot quickly retrieve the needed word. In either case, the script will lack elaboration and detail. Basically, the child's script will sound very general and vague.
- Children with language impairment may have difficulty expressing the temporal or causal organization required for script telling. Many children, even "normally developing" children have difficulty with relational terms and causal constructions such as "because" and "if/then." The most frequently used conjunction ("and") may not indicate full understanding of the temporal or causal relationship in the script.
- Some children have a great deal of difficulty making the narrative hold together for a listener. The child may go off on tangents or lose the main idea of the narrative, even though focused questions demonstrate that the child understands the temporal or causal relationships in the narrative.
- The child may have an inefficient processing system. As a result. the child can only retrieve the script slowly or may have difficulty maintaining or changing the script as needed. The narrative shows response delays, difficulty changing tasks, and the need for repetitions and cues.
- The child may have difficulties with the advance planning of the account and difficulties self-monitoring the adequacy of what is said as he or she goes along. The outcome is a series of sentences that are not organized in a coherent systematic manner. The child has difficulty moving from talking about a personal experience to a more generalized account.

- It should be considered that the child might not have had sufficient experience with the event to have developed a script. We do not know how many exposures to an experience a child with language impairment needs to develop script knowledge. To rule out this possibility, the clinician can back up to the nonverbal task of acting out, or arranging pictures, or observing the child in the situation.

Assessing Personal Event Narratives

Unlike the script telling discussed previously, a personal narrative is the telling of a particular event or experience. A good personal narrative has a point. That is to say, there is a particular reason for telling about the event. For example, telling about a time that you were very frightened, or telling about a funny thing that happened on your family vacation. Personal narratives use first person pronouns ("I", "we") and

> In contrast to scripts, the topic or foreground of a personal narrative is the unfolding of a particular episode and general event information is only provided as commentary or background information.
> Hudson and Shapiro (1995), p. 95

past tense constructions. The personal narrative is organized around a high point, which is the point of the narrative.

By 6 years old, a child can tell a well-formed personal narrative that orients a listener to who, what, and where something happened. The narrative includes a sequence of events that build to a climax or high point and then resolves by telling how things turned out. (McCabe & Rollins, 1994)

How can the SLP assess personal narrative ability?

It is most appropriate with young children to use a real past event as the catalyst for the personal narrative. We suggest beginning with a demonstration of a personal narrative or a prompt for the narrative. The exact content of this demonstration is not important. It is important that the child hear an appropriate personal narrative that builds to a climax.

Example Demonstration

Have you ever been camping? One time when I was your age I went camping with my family. The first night we were putting up the tent and found out that Dad forgot the center pole at home. It was getting very dark, so my dad went into the woods and cut down a small tree. The little tree held up the tent until it started to rain real hard at night. It was so dark and there was thunder and lightning. The roof of the tent started to fall in because the little tree was bending. My brother and sister and I were getting so wet and so scared we didn't know what to do. We started to yell for Dad, who was in the car. We yelled and yelled and my little sister was crying because she was scared. Pretty soon, Dad heard us and he went to the woods again and got another tree. This one was stronger and it held the tent up for the whole rest of the trip.

Instruction

In general most children will tell the best stories about being hurt or scared. After telling your story, ask the child to tell about a time he or she was scared or hurt. Or ask the child to tell you about a funny thing that happened on a trip that was made with his family (especially if you know that the child went somewhere unusual).

It is a good idea to collect at least three narratives from a child. No prompt is going to work equally well with every child. By asking for three narratives, you are increasing the chances of striking on something that the child really wants to talk about.

Responding

Children are used to telling personal narratives to a listener who responds and it is through such responses that the narrative grows. Clinicians need to respond, also. It is important that the nature of the response encourages narration without directing it. In general, responses should be generic. Try repeating the exact words that the child just said. This encourages the child by showing him that you are listening and are interested. Say things like "uh-huh" or "Tell me more" or "Then what." All of these things said with inflection and facial expression that conveys interest in the child and the story will encourage the child to expand. It is important to avoid saying too much. The more the clinician talks, the less the child will. The more evaluative our statements seem to the child, the less he or she will be willing to share with us. Be sure not to rush a child. For many reasons, it is important to take the time to listen to the child's narrative. (McCabe & Rollins, 1994)

Examples of Personal Narratives

All of these narratives were gathered after determining conversationally that the child takes family trips.

> **Example 1**—This is an example of a well-constructed narrative. Note the use of personal pronouns (I) and past tense verbs. There is background information telling who, when, and where the event took place. There is a clear high point (the brother "threw up all over the seat . . ."), there is a resolution ("leave the windows open"), and there is an evaluation ("we got really cold").
>
> **Adult:** Tell me about one time when your family took a trip.
>
> **Child:** One time we went to my grandma's house for Christmas, and my dad was driving and my mom was in the front seat. I was in the back with my

little brother. We were just driving along, and all of a sudden he threw up all over the seat and the floor and everywhere. My dad had to stop and my mom cleaned up all the mess, but the car smelled so bad we had to leave the windows open and we got really cold.

Example 2—This is not a personal narrative. It is more like a list of events. It lacks a high point.

Adult: Tell me about one time when your family took a trip.

Child: We went to Disney World, and we went on the rides and we got to swim in the pool at the motel and we went to the restaurant.

Example 3—This narrative has less coherent organization. That is, the things that happen are not in any particular order. There is however a high point (sunburn) and an evaluation ("it really hurt").

Adult: Tell me about one time when your family took a trip.

Child: We went to the ocean. First we had to go on the airplane, then we drove to my cousin's house. Then everyday we went to the beach and we looked for shells and stuff, and waded in the water. And I got a sunburn and my mom had to put stuff all on my back and my arms and everywhere, and it really hurt.

How can the SLP evaluate a personal narrative?

There are five things to look for in the transcript of a child's personal narrative.

- Does the child use an appropriate personal pronoun (I, we)? In general, does the child use the past tense?
- Does the student have some kind of introducer? For young children this might be, "You know what". For older children it will be a statement that picks up on your prompt such as "I got hurt when . . ."
- Does the child provide background and setting information? "Last summer we went to . . ."
- Is there a high point to the narrative? Are there actions leading to the high point? Does the high point include an evaluation by the child, for example "I was scared."
- Is there an ending to the narrative that resolves the complications or high point?

How are the results interpreted?

As has been discussed several times in this book, it is impossible to rate any given child's personal narrative skills without having an idea what other children of similar experience would provide in the same context.

The most important distinguishing feature of the personal narrative is the presence of a high point. If the child does not include a high point, then the child is not providing you with a personal narrative. If it can be assumed that the topic was something that most children would provide a personal narrative for and that this child has had this experience, then we can assume that the child is not capable of providing a personal narrative.

If the child does provide a high point but does not provide background information or does not draw the narrative to a close, then we can assume that the student has the experience to provide the narrative and some idea of the structural requirements of a narrative, but lacks the elaboration skills required to provide a complete narrative.

If a child demonstrates the use of the personal narrative structure (includes a high point), but does not use the appropriate verb form, we would not consider this to be a problem with understanding and using the personal narrative structure.

Assessing Story Structure

What is story structure?

Story structure, or framework, is another type of narrative. The story framework is a mental representation of a story. Children use the framework as a "hook" on which to hang new stories that they hear, read, or originate. In this sense then, the pres-

> While scripts are schemata formed in the child's mind based on experiences with the real world, story frameworks are dictated by stories themselves.

ence of a story structure and a child's ability to use it will aid the child in reading comprehension.

The use of a story framework appears to be universal, but the particular structure of the framework is culturally determined by the nature of stories within a given culture. The story structure discussed in this section comes from a Western European tradition. Within this tradition stories are made up of characters, a setting, a plot, and an ending. The plot consists of a series of episodes. Research has demonstrated that an episode is the focal point of story framework and it is the knowledge of the structure of an episode that has been found to be the best predictor of the child's future reading comprehension success (Fazio et al., 1996).

What is an episode?

The episode is that part of a story that moves the plot along. It is the part of the story that teachers refer to as "the middle" when they are teaching children how to write stories. The episode has three parts:

- The *initiating event* (IE), which is some event (internal or external) that causes a disequilibrium for the character;

- The *attempt* (A), which is the character's response or attempt to deal with the disequilibrium;
- The *consequence* (C), which is the outcome of the character's attempt.

How does story structure develop?

It is clear that understanding and use of underlying story structure develops over time. Most children develop a story framework, because they have been read to during the first 5 years of life. At first, the best books for very young children have very clear episodic structure, with all three parts of each episode clearly depicted. However as the stories become more complex as the child ages, frequently parts of an episode are left to be inferred by the child through the use of world knowledge. It is not until fifth grade that children can tell coherent, goal-based, original stories. However children as young as kindergarten can demonstrate the understanding of story framework through story retelling tasks.

How is story structure assessed?

The best way to assess story structure is by eliciting a story-retelling. Using story retelling allows us to provide the child with the additional support of the story being told and using the pictures in the story to support the retelling. If the story chosen takes into account the child's world knowledge (script), this also provides more support. All of these supports lighten the processing load for the student.

How is story retelling assessed?

- The first consideration is the choice of a book. Fazio et.al. (1996) demonstrated that if a chosen story was based on a familiar childhood script (e.g., going to bed) the child's knowledge of the script supports his or her story structure knowledge, which results in better retelling. In other words, the research indicates that story-retelling performance is influenced by a child's knowledge of the content of a story. The more a story draws on the child's world knowledge, the better the story retelling will be. The younger the child, the more important it is that the book be based on a script that the child knows
- The clarity of the episodic structure is very important when choosing a book for assessment. The book should contain five or six episodes. The parts of each episode should be very clearly stated. It is not unusual for an initiating event to be implied after the initial statement and it is also not unusual for either the attempt or the consequence to be implied. If all three parts of each episode are not transparently clear, the clinician will have to fill in those parts before reading the story to the child.
- The third issue to consider is the pictures. As it is the pictures that will guide and support a child's retelling, it is vitally important that the pictures clearly represent each part of an episode. If there is no pictorial representation of a part of an episode, then if a child leaves out that part, it will be very difficult to know whether the child just forgot or whether the part is missing as a piece of his or her story framework.

The following two books are examples of the type to be used in assessment: *Timothy and the Night Noises* by Jeffrey Dinardo and *My Tooth is Loose!* by Martin Silverman. Both of these books fulfill the requirements. They are script based, they are 5 or 6 episodes long, and the pictures correspond wonderfully with the parts of each episode.

Materials

When the book has been chosen, a score sheet must be prepared. Initially each episode and each part of each episode is identified. Each episode is then paraphrased onto the score sheet with short designations for each part of the episode (see example score sheet in Appendix 5D at the end of this chapter). It is important to paraphrase or use key words, so we do not forget that a child is encouraged to use personal words in the retelling.

The text of the book must be covered, so that the child will not be tempted to try to read the story. Copy the text of the book on a separate sheet of paper that you will use to "read" the book during the task administration.

Administration

To administer this task, sit next to the child so that we can "share" the book. Carefully place the book squarely in front of the child so that he or she can clearly see the pictures and is able to follow along with the story.

You will want to begin by introducing the story to the child to help the student bring his or her world knowledge/script knowledge to bear on listening to the story. For example:

> Introduction for *Timothy and the Night Noises*: "This is a story about a frog who is afraid of the dark. I'll bet you know someone who is afraid of the dark."

> Introduction for *My Tooth is Loose*! "This is a story about a boy with a loose tooth and he doesn't know what to do. I'll bet you have had a loose tooth."

Instructions

"I will **tell** you the story, then you look at the pictures and tell the story into my tape recorder." It is recommended that you use the word "tell" rather than read, so as not to raise a child's anxiety about being asked to read.

Tell the story slowly and with expression. Point to the important parts of the pictures such as which character you are talking about or some important occurrence in the story. This part of the task should be very similar to any joint adult/child reading activity. Give the child plenty of time to look at the pictures and comment. It is important during this aspect of the task to remember that children with language impairment frequently have a slower language processing time.

When the story is completed, give the child the book and tell him or her to tell the story. Children should be encouraged to use their own words. Frequently children need help to get started. It is not unusual for a child to hesitate in the beginning, because he or she does not remember the character's names. With *Timothy and the Night Noises,* we usually start out by saying, "Now you tell me about Timothy and Martin," as we point to each of them. Because the names of the characters are not the important part of the episodic structure, a child can call the characters any name. This frequently happens with *My Tooth Is Loose!* because there are many children in the story.

You may prompt a child as much as necessary through the initial setting of the story. As soon as the first episode begins (see score sheet), you must refrain from prompts other than "then what" or "tell me more." Do not say "tell me about this picture/page," because that will generally encourage a child to describe the picture.

Recording Responses

- To begin the analysis process, transcribe the child's retelling, verbatim, from the tape. It is not necessary to transcribe your prompts, as long as they were the generic "tell me more" or "then what." With practice, you will find that you can transcribe directly onto the score sheet.
- Using a score sheet (see example in Appendix 5D), transfer the child's retelling to the appropriate area on the score sheet.
- The episodes do not necessarily need to be told in order.
- The parts of an episode do not have to be told in order; for example, the child may tell the consequence and then the attempt.
- However, the initiating event-attempt-consequence must all be from the same episode and told together for the episode to count. In other words, the child can not tell the attempt from Episode 2 while trying to tell Episode 1 and have it count for either episode.
- On the score sheet, you will notice that there are several initiating event statements, attempt statements, and consequence statements for each episode. These are optional ways of fulfilling the requirement for each part of an episode. A child needs to give just one of the options to get credit for that part of the episode.
- A child does not need to use the same words or say things exactly as you read a story. When a child uses his or her own words, it indicates that the child has stored the meaning of the text and if the student uses the episodic structure it indicates that the child uses this style of structure to support the storage or retrieval of the stored meaning.
- Other errors that may be noted in the transcript, such as verb tense, morphological endings, pronoun confusions, and syntax are not part of the story structure analysis.
- When you have finished scoring you indicate how many complete episodes were retold. The criterion we have been using based on Fazio et al. (1996) and our local norms is that a child who could retell half the episodes (i.e., 3/5) demonstrated adequate story structure. This criterion is based on the two books mentioned. Needless to say, if different books are chosen, it will be necessary to establish local norms for those particular books. Refer to the section of this book that discusses criterion-referenced testing and establishing local norms.

- If a child does not meet the recommended criterion, it is necessary to analyze the retelling to determine what parts of the episodes the child did or did not retell. The analysis of the episode parts provides a basis for intervention procedures.
- Following this analysis, we consider why a child is not using a mental representation—a story structure. As the assessment of narrative skills is only part of the total assessment, the answers may come from other assessment protocols. If a child does not use a story structure, it may be because the child:
    a. Lacks sufficient background knowledge about the narrative topic;
    b. Has a word-finding difficulty;
    c. Has inadequate vocabulary—especially the vocabulary that holds or ties the episodic structure together;
    d. Processes language inefficiently—that is, has difficulty converting self-knowledge of story structure into linguistic units.

Sample Story Retelling Scoring

Sample #1

6 yrs, 4 mos. 1st grade

Total Episode: 1/5

It is your bedtime, Timothy and Martin	**Setting**	
Timothy put on his pajamas.	**Setting**	
He kissed both of them.	**Setting**	
He heard a WOOO	**Initiating Event**	**Episode #1**
He say Mama	**Attempt**	"
It only the wind, Martin	**Consequence**	"

Sample #2

6 yrs, 6 mos. 1st grade

Total Episode: 0 /5

It is the bedtime	**Setting**	
He put on his p.j.s	**Setting**	
She said go to bed.	**Setting**	
Martin heard a ghost.	**Initiating Event**	**Episode #1**
Martin jumped out of bed	**Attempt**	**Episode #2**
It's only the tree, Martin	**Consequence**	**Episode #3**
Martin heard a peck on his head	**Initiating Event**	**Episode #5**
OOOO	**Initiating Event**	**Episode #5**
The end	**Ending**	

How are narrative skills discussed at the IEP conference?

- The child's ability to understand and put into words what he or she has experienced has a profound affect on his ability to understand, remember, and discuss the experiences a character has in a story that the class reads.
- The child's ability to discuss and answer questions about stories the student has heard or read is how teachers assess the child's reading comprehension abilities.
- Having a framework for narration, whether it is in the form of script, personal narrative, or story, allows the child to store what he or she hears or reads. If the child has a framework to "hang" the story on, the child can use most of his energy to answer questions about the text or write a story. If the child does not have such a framework or cannot access the framework, then the story that he or she has read and is asked to discuss is just so many unrelated sentences that the student is trying to recall. This results in a heavy processing load. The more one has to juggle at once, the more difficult a task becomes. You might use the analogy of driving a car. In learning to drive a car, you had to concentrate on every movement; as you gained skill and competence, you could drive and eat, and talk, and switch the cassettes in the tape player at the same time.
- Based on the results of the total assessment, it is recommended that the child engage in activities to facilitate the use of script-knowledge or story-retelling skills, not as ends in themselves but as an aid to reading and listening comprehension skills.

Summary

Narrative assessment is not intended to determine *if* a child has language impairment. The benefit of using a narrative assessment is to help you identify needed areas of intervention for a child with language impairment.

The underlying issue with narrative abilities is processing load. Narrative abilities are important because, with good use of them, a child can use all of his or her cognitive energy to concentrate on new information required for completing classroom activities (i.e., answering comprehension questions).

Assessment of narration is a criterion-referenced task and, as such, needs to be considered in light of what is required in a child's classroom and how other children in the classroom complete the same task.

With narrative assessment completed and interpreted, clinicians can now move to establishing goals and developing intervention strategies.

APPENDIX 5A

Checklist for Script Assessment

☐ Determine the child's experiences and choose a script from among those experienced by the child.

☐ Determine appropriate level to begin the assessment:

    ☐ Act out the script with manipulatives

    ☐ Arrange pictures depicting the script

    ☐ Give a verbal account of an event

☐ Transcribe the child's script verbatim and analyze it compared to other children from the same grade and experience level.

    ☐ Did the child use "you" in the script telling?

    ☐ Did the child use the present tense in the retelling?

    ☐ Did the child use temporal, spatial, and/or causal organizational devices in the retelling?

APPENDIX 5B

Checklist for Personal Event Narrative

☐ Demonstrate an event narrative by telling one yourself.

☐ Determine something that has happened in the child's life that will elicit this style of narrative.

☐ Gather at least 2 event narratives from the child

☐ Transcribe the narratives verbatim and compare them to narratives given by other children in the same grade.

☐ Analyze the transcript:

　　☐ Did the child use the personal pronoun (I, we)?

　　☐ Did the child generally use the past tense?

　　☐ Did the child use a mechanism for introducing the narrative?

　　☐ Did the child provide background/setting information?

　　☐ Does the narrative contain a high point?

　　☐ Does the narrative include an ending that resolves the complications or high point?

APPENDIX 5C

Story Retelling Score Sheet
for *Timothy and the Night Noises*

Name _____ School _____

Grade _____ Date _____ Number of episodes told _____/5

Instructions

Transcribe the child's retelling. From the transcript, fill in the parts of the episodes on this form. The child does not have to give the exact text and the child does not have to give the elements in book order. In the space provided, record how many complete episodes the child retold. If the child did not tell at least three (3) complete episodes, analyze which parts of the episodes the child did tell. The setting and ending parts of the story are not scored.

Setting

It was late (or bedtime). Timothy, Martin, Mama Martin put on his pajamas. He had a little trouble. He hopped into bed. Mama tucked them in. She kissed them good night. Timothy said, "I'm scared." He wants the light on. Mama said he's a big boy (frog) now. There's nothing to be afraid of Martin is here. Martin rolled over. Mama turned off the light. She left the room. Timothy asked Martin if he'd really protect him. Martin told him not to be a fathead.

Episode 1

Timothy heard a noise	IE
WOOO	IE
Mama help me	A
Said heard a ghost	A
Mama came in	C
It was only the wind	C
Martin rolled his eyes	C
Mama tucked him in	C
Mama sat for awhile	C
Timothy tried to sleep	C
Timothy closed his eyes	C

Episode 2

He heard a noise	IE
Creak, creak	IE
He jumped into Mama's lap	A
"What's that?"	A
It's only the chair	C
Timothy rocked the chair	C

Episode 3

He saw something moving	IE
He said it was a monster	A
It's the shadow of a tree	C
Mama tucked him in	C
Mama left the room	C

Episode 4

Martin said Timothy was a baby	IE
Timothy said he wasn't	A
Martin made a face and rolled over	C

Episode 5

Martin felt something tap him on the shoulder	IE
BOOO	IE
Martin said "AHH, a ghost"	A
He ran out of the room	A
He returned with mama	C
Mama said there's no ghost	C
She tucked Martin in	C
She looked at Timothy	C

Ending

He was asleep

APPENDIX 5D

Story Retelling Score Sheet
for *My Tooth is Loose*!

Name _____ School _____

Grade _____ Date _____ Number of episodes told _____/6

Instructions

Transcribe the child's retelling. From the transcript, fill in the parts of the episodes on this form. The child does not have to give the exact text nor does the child have to give the elements in order. Record how many complete episodes were retold in the space provided. If the child did not tell at least three (3) complete episodes, analyze which parts of the episodes the child did tell. The setting part of the story is not scored.

Setting

He wasn't playing. He just sat there. "What's wrong?"

Episode 1

My tooth is loose	IE
I don't know what to do	IE
Dad took mine out witha string	A
Don't want a string	C

Episode 2

Tooth is loose	IE
Don't know what to do	IE
Bite apple	A
Don't want to bite apple	C
Might hurt	C

Episode 3

Tooth is loose	IE
Don't know what to do	IE
Dentist pull it	A
Don't want the dentist	C

Episode 4

Tooth is loose	IE
Don't know what to do	IE
Twist it	A
Won't twist it	C
Might bleed	C

Episode 5

Tooth is loose	IE
Grandma gave me fudge	A
Swallowed my tooth	A
Don't want to swallow	C
Might grow inside	C

Episode 6

Mama, tooth is loose	IE
Open your mouth	A
Let me look at your tooth	A
Don't touch	A
You don't have to do anything	A
Tooth will come out by itself	A
And it did	C

CHAPTER

6

Intervention for Narrative Skills

Principles of Narrative Intervention

1. Acknowledge the role of first- and second-hand experience in the development of narrative frameworks such as scripts and story grammars.

2. Recognize cultural differences in scripted event knowledge and story structure.

3. Acknowledge the developmental nature of personal event narratives in young children.

4. Facilitate development of narrative abilities in school-age children using stories based on familiar scripted events and organized around a culturally significant story framework.

5. Use assessment results to develop measurable goals and objectives and to determine where to begin intervention.

6. Mediate for students to give them a purpose for developing narrative skills.

7. Understand it is never too late to start.

8. Introduce concepts to teachers, administrators, and parents.

9. Integrate concepts into the language arts curriculum for all students at the early elementary level (K–3).

Taking A Closer Look

Principle #1: Acknowledge the role of first- and second-hand experience in the development of narrative frameworks such as scripts and story grammars.

- Narratives are mapped onto knowledge about the world that comes from experience.
- Children with limited experiences may have fewer or less-detailed scripts.
- Students should be asked to recount events that they have directly experienced or at least been told or read to about.
- Parents, siblings, teachers, and classmates need to be employed as resources when determining the nature and extent of a student's experience with an event.
- Books chosen for intervention activities should be based on familiar scripted events.

Principle #2: Recognize cultural differences in scripted event knowledge and story structure.

- Some experiences are culturally specific. A clinician needs to be cautious about interpreting the accuracy of an event recount based on an experience with which he or she is not familiar.
- Some experiences are crosscultural, but the details of the events are variable, according to family tradition or lifestyle.

Principle #3: Acknowledge the developmental nature of personal event narratives in young children.

- Develop goals and objectives that reflect the developmental nature of narrative abilities.
- Regardless of a child's chronological age, follow the developmental sequence for developing narrative abilities.
- Implement lessons that encourage conversation about real past events that are important to young children, such as "getting hurt" or experiencing a misfortune.
- Plan activities that provide opportunities for conversation about real experiences.

Principle #4: Facilitate development of narrative abilities in school-age children, using stories based on familiar scripted events and organized around culturally significant story frameworks.

- Choose episodic stories based on familiar scripted events for intervention with most North American, English-speaking children.
- Select stories in which the pictures clearly support the episodes.
- Make sure that stories with multiple episodes are clearly sequenced.
- Episodic stories used for intervention should be of appropriate length and linguistic complexity.
- Pretest stories through clinician retelling.

Principle #5: Use assessment results to develop measurable goals and objectives and to determine where to begin intervention.

- Select assessment tools that diagnose what the student **can do** as well as what the student needs to learn.
- Assess early narrative abilities, if later developing skills are missing.
- Develop goals and objectives that reflect a student's performance on meaningful measures of narrative assessment.
- Begin intervention with all students, regardless of age, based on performance levels determined by assessment.

Principle #6: Mediate for students to give them a purpose for developing narrative skills.

- The connection between developing narrative skills and learning to read and write is not obvious to students and, thus, needs to be explained.
- Explain the relationship between narrative skills and literacy once or twice in simple terms. Then begin each intervention lesson with a brief reminder that narrative skills will help students to improve reading and writing skills.
- Mediate to motivate students to learn difficult concepts. It gives them a real purpose for learning.
- Provide students with opportunities to appreciate each of their accomplishments as they work toward learning to retell events and stories.

Principle #7: Understand that it is never too late to start narrative intervention.

- We have successfully used narrative intervention activities with students from age 3 years through age 12.
- We have observed selected students with mild-to-moderate developmental disabilities benefit from narrative intervention.
- Narrative intervention activities can be appropriately modified using picture symbols for the nonspeaking population.

Principle #8: Introduce concepts to teachers, administrators, and parents.

- Report on narrative abilities in diagnostic reports to be shared at case conferences.
- Share research with other professionals through in-services.
- Enlist the help of others in establishing local norms for story retelling.
- Model instructional techniques for teachers and support staff.
- Inform parents about narrative development by making a presentation at a parent meeting.

Principle #9: Integrate concepts into the language arts curriculum for all students at the early elementary level (K–3).

- Participate in revisions of the language arts curriculum in your school district. A speech-language pathologist who understands the role narrative development plays in reading comprehension can be a valuable asset on a language arts curriculum committee.

- Participate in textbook adoption. Help find materials for early elementary students that include stories based on familiar scripted events with clear episodic structure.
- Advocate for early elementary teachers to have access to a variety of materials for developing early narrative skills within the classroom setting.
- Participate in activities such as field trips, hands-on classroom experiences, daily routines, and reading aloud that clearly support development of narrative skills.

Narrative Goals and Objectives

We have developed goals and objectives for teaching production of early narrative skills, as well as using narrative frameworks to support increased performance in reading comprehension and written language. Our list demonstrates how goals and objectives for narration can be written in an academically relevant manner. We often use the list during conferences to educate parents and teachers about the relationship between narrative development and language arts proficiencies at the early, middle, and late elementary levels.

Goal

The student will increase expressive language skills by using narrative frameworks to structure production of oral narratives.

Objectives

- To act out scripts for generalized events.
- To use language to compose accounts of generalized event scripts.
- To use generalized event scripts to structure verbal accounts of personally experienced events.
- To retell "initiating events" within simple episodic stories.
- To retell "attempts" within simple episodic stories.
- To retell "consequences" within simple episodic stories.
- To retell one complete episode within an episodic story.
- To retell half of the episodes within an episodic story.

Goal

The student will increase receptive language skills by using narrative frameworks to structure comprehension of narratives read or heard.

Objectives

- To tell the setting of a story.
- To tell the main characters of a story.
- To give accurate answers to questions about an episode of a story.
- To give logical answers to inferential questions about an episode of a story.
- To determine the plot of an episodic story.

- To give accurate answers to questions about the plot of a story.
- To give logical answers to inferential questions about the plot of a story.

Goal

The student will increase written language skills by using narrative frameworks to structure production of written narratives.

Objectives

- To plan an episode, given 2 out of 3 parts.
- To plan an episode, given 1 out of 3 parts.
- To plan an episode that extends a story.
- To plan 2 episodes which extend a story.
- To plan an original story with 1 episode.
- To plan an original story with 2 episodes.
- To draft an episode, given 2 out of 3 parts.
- To draft an episode, given 1 out of 3 parts.
- To draft an episode that extends a story.
- To draft 2 episodes that extend a story.
- To draft an original story with 1 episode.
- To draft an original story with 2 episodes.
- To write an episode, given 2 out of 3 parts.
- To write an episode, given 1 out of 3 parts.
- To write an episode that extends a story.
- To write 2 episodes that extend a story.
- To write an original story with 1 episode.
- To write an original story with 2 episodes.

A Word About Our Lesson Plans for Narrative Skills Intervention

Our goal in this section is to prepare you to begin narrative intervention with students who demonstrate limited ability to recount familiar events, comprehend episodic stories, and retell episodic stories. The following lesson plans may be used for individual or group activities. Examples of group activities are given occasionally, simply because many clinicians find them difficult to plan. We hope that clinicians will find this section helpful as they collaborate with special education and general education teachers. The sample lesson plans provided include valuable information meant to be shared with all those committed to improving the language arts skills of students with language impairment. Some clinicians may even find selected lessons appropriate for sharing with interested parents.

Each lesson plan includes:

1. Introduction to procedures.
2. Objectives for each lesson.
3. Materials needed.

4. Basic clinician script.

5. Student script.

6. Suggested cueing strategies.

7. Suggested criteria for mastery for each lesson.

Taking a Closer Look

The **introduction** for each lesson includes a reminder of its clinical and educational relevance. It describes the role of the clinician, teachers, and parents in developing a particular skill. It also suggests various intervention contexts that have proved successful in our experience.

The **objectives** for each lesson are presented in simple form. They should be made measurable by the case conference team through adding context and criteria. We realize that some districts insist that progress be reported strictly in terms of percentages; others acknowledge that reporting gains in terms of the amount of support a child needs to maintain performance levels similar to those of their peers is more meaningful.

Materials needed for each lesson are listed. Most are easily made or attainable at a local teacher supply store or craft store. The children's books listed are currently in print and should be available at a local library, bookstore, or online book vendor. We are frequently asked about using intervention "kits." We do not use kits to teach narrative skills. We use only the materials listed in the lesson plans.

A **basic clinician script** for each lesson is outlined to give clinicians, teachers, and parents a general idea of what we say to our students as we proceed through each lesson. It is not meant to be "the only way" to talk with the students, but should give an indication of our approach. Remember, mediation is a powerful communication tool, as well as self-talk. Be sure that students know the purpose of each activity, and that thinking strategies are verbalized during demonstrations.

A **student script** for each lesson is provided to give clinicians, teachers, and parents an idea what students say or do when their responses are "on the right track." The scripts are based on our observations of students while learning specific concepts.

Suggested cueing strategies are described because of the importance of providing scaffolding throughout the intervention process. The cues provided are taken directly from our clinical and classroom experiences with students. They vary in nature and intensity depending on the student's response to a given learning opportunity. If students seem to rely too heavily on cues, consider the need for additional demonstration or teaching.

Suggested criteria for mastery of specific concepts are outlined for each lesson. We generally recommend reaching a mastery level of performance before proceeding to the next lesson. However, in special cases in which mastery learning is not a realistic expectation, criteria for moving to the next lesson may need to be set on an individual basis. Under these circumstances, frequent review of previously "learned" concepts through direct practice and mediation is the key to successful intervention.

Lesson Plans for Narrative Skills Intervention

Teaching About Scripts: Demonstrating Scripted Events

Introduction

Some children need help learning how to act out events with props or through role-playing. For others, arranging a set of pictures to represent important parts of the event may be a more appropriate way to begin intervention. Each of these activities provides an opportunity for a child to demonstrate the ability to access a familiar script before being asked to put the script into language.

Parents, caregivers, and teachers should be the primary sources of information when determining the types of events a student has experienced. Although most children have had experiences with scripted events, such as getting ready for bed, going to the doctor, and having a birthday party, specific information about a child's world knowledge is best gathered through interviews or written questionnaires.

Objectives

There is one basic objective for teaching beginning narrative skill. The child must show access to generalized event scripts through acting out generalized events using props and role-playing or through picture arrangement. Remember, this step can be omitted if assessment shows the ability to act out generalized events is intact.

Materials

Manipulatives such as props or pictures associated with the script that the student is going to act out should be provided.

Clinician Script

The clinician must remember to set up the scenario to be acted out. For example, "I have been invited to a birthday party tomorrow. I'm a little worried, because I don't know what to do at a birthday party. I've never been to one before. " The clinician then tells the child to use provided toys to show what happens at a birthday party. Remember to note the child's ability to use pretend play, in general. A 4-year-old who lacks pretend play skills is really not developmentally ready to act out event scripts.

If a picture arrangement task is used instead of acting out the event, the setup is much the same. But as this is an artificial task, devoid of context, a reason should be provided for completing the task similar to the example given above.

Student Script

The student either acts out the event using props provided by the clinician or arranges pictures that represent the parts of the event in a logical order.

Suggested Cueing Strategies

Cueing strategies such as, "Show me what happens *first.*" are often used to get a child started. Additional cues such as, "Show me what happens *next/last*" can also be helpful if, in fact, the child can demonstrate the event script. Offering to help by saying, "I think I remember what happens *after that*" followed by a model can be beneficial as a child is learning the task.

Suggested Criteria for Mastery

Once a child has demonstrated the ability to consistently access generalized event scripts through nonverbal demonstration, mastery is suggested.

Lesson Plan: Demonstrating Scripted Events

Objective

To act out scripts for generalized events.

Materials

Props suitable for acting out or role-playing a given scripted event or pictures that, when arranged properly, represent the event.

Activity

Students act out a given scripted event for which the clinician has determined there is significant experience or arranges pictures in a logical order to represent the event.

Procedures: Demonstration of the Event

Demonstration: Mediation should inform the student that the clinician is aware of the child's experience with a particular scripted event. For example, "I was talking to your mom the other day and she said you know all about fishing. I don't know about fishing, but I know about birthdays. I am going to use these toys and show you all I know about birthdays." The clinician proceeds to act out a birthday party using props. In this case, the props consist of flannel board pieces (invitations, people, presents, cake, ice cream, etc.)

- ○ **Clinician:** "My uncle is taking me fishing this weekend. I need to learn all I can about fishing right away! Show me what happens when you go fishing. Use the toys/pictures to help you."

- ○ **Student:** Student uses props to act out event in an organized, logical manner that demonstrates sufficient knowledge of the generalized event.

- ○ **Clinician:** Provide cues as needed to help the student act out the event.

Teaching About Scripts: Narrating Generalized Event Scripts

Introduction

The next step in teaching scripted event recounting is to help students with language impairment to convert familiar generalized event scripts into linguistic form. Although still an artificial task, providing opportunities for students to compose verbal accounts of generalized events is a necessary step in teaching narrative skills.

Objectives

The ability to use language to talk about generalized scripted events should be demonstrated before asking a child to use language to give a verbal account of a personal experience. In general, scripted events that are temporally sequenced are the easiest for young children and those with cognitive impairments to recount. Once mastered, using language to structure accounts of generalized events that are causally related should be the focus.

Materials

As in the assessment task, no specific materials are required. However, we find it helpful to have a general picture of an event to provide a reason for asking for the script.

Clinician's Role

The clinician should provide students with an understanding of who the audience for the narrative might be and set a purpose for communicating the information to be shared. This decreases the artificiality of the therapy situation. In other words, give the student a reason for telling a specific person or group of people about a scripted event. At school, we try to use realistic scenarios such as a new student in the classroom, eating lunch at school, or participating in a school program.

Student's Role

The student plays an active role by using language to tell about the generalized scripted event as completely and coherently as possible.

Suggested Cueing Strategies

Cueing strategies such as "Tell me what happens *first*" are often used to get a child started telling temporally ordered events. Additional cues such as, "Tell me what happens *next/last*" can also be helpful if a child loses focus for any reason. Offering to help by saying, "I know what happens *after that*" followed by providing a model can be beneficial for a child just beginning to learn the task. Causally ordered events can be cued with "*What if*" questions that invite elaboration and additional detail.

Suggested Criteria for Mastery

Assuming that previous assessment revealed inadequacies in a student's script telling ability when compared to other children in the child's classroom, mastery would be reached when these differences no longer exist. However, we realize that, for some students with language impairment, performing at a level commensurate with same age peers is an unrealistic goal. For these students we suggest that the script telling should at least contain the word "you" and show logical temporal and/or causal organization.

Lesson Plan: Narrating Generalized Event Scripts

Objective

To use language to tell generalized event scripts.

Materials

Props are not required, but a picture or prop that represents an important part of the scripted event helps students focus.

Activity

Students tell about a scripted event for which the clinician has determined adequate world knowledge exists.

Procedures

Narration of the event.

Demonstration: Mediation should inform the student that the clinician is aware of the child's experience with a particular scripted event. For example, "I was talking to your mom the other day and she said you know all about fishing. I don't know about fishing, but I know about birthdays. I am going to use these toys and tell you all I know about birthdays." The clinician proceeds to tell about parties using props. In this case, the props consist of flannel board pieces (invitations, people, presents, cake, ice cream, etc.)

- ○ **Clinician:** "Tell me what you know about _____. Use the toys/pictures to help you."
- ○ **Student:** Student uses props to act out scripted event in a manner that demonstrates temporal and or causal organization.
- ○ **Clinician:** Provides cues as needed to help the student organize the telling of the generalized event script as needed.

Teaching About Personal Narratives: Telling Personal Events

Introduction

Using language to tell about personal events and experiences in a logical, organized, coherent manner is vital to school success. Children call on this narrative framework to communicate with parents about classroom events and share family experiences with teachers and friends. We must create repeated opportunities for students with language impairment to practice relating personal events and experiences. Without this early developing narrative skill under their belts, students with language disorders will continue to struggle with comprehension of stories read and heard throughout their school careers.

Objectives

There is one basic objective for teaching about personal event narratives. Students need to be taught to use generalized event scripts to structure their verbal accounts of personally experienced events. The result will be a personal narrative organized around a high point that satisfies the purpose for telling about the experience.

Materials

For some children no materials are needed. Conversation about familiar topics will remind them of personal experiences to tell about, even though their account of the personal experience lacks structure and or content. For other children, particularly those with cognitive delays, memory issues, or word-finding problems, children's books based on familiar scripts should be used to remind them that they have relevant personal experiences to share.

Clinician's Role

The clinician's role is to create a context for telling personal narratives that make sense. The personal narratives should be based on familiar scripted events, such as going camping or visiting grandma's house. The clinician should use scaffolding techniques to help students tell about experiences before asking them to recount them independently. Demonstration is an important step for many students, because they need opportunities to hear how personal event narratives are organized. Personal experiences recounted by the clinician should be based on familiar scripted events such as going camping or visiting grandma's house. When it is time for the students to begin telling their own personal narratives, the clinician should use scaffolding techniques to assure that the event sequence builds to a high point followed by a resolution.

Student's Role

The student attends to the clinician's demonstrations and attempts to tell about personal experiences based on real past events. If students are participating in small group therapy sessions, they need to know there is a purpose for listening to the personal narratives.

Suggested Cueing Strategies

The type of cueing strategies used to support the telling of a personal event narrative is dependent on the organization and coherence of the narrative told. General forms of encouragement such as "Uh-huh" or "Tell me more" or "Then what" show the student that you are listening and interested and not considered clinically significant support cues.

Suggested Criteria for Mastery

A student who tells personal event narratives that include the personal pronouns "I" and "we," use of the past tense, and a statement that acts as an introducer has mastered the structural components of the personal event narrative. A student who provides background and setting information, a high point with actions leading up to it, an evaluation of the high point, and an ending to the narrative that resolves the complications or high point, tells a personal event narrative that includes appropriate content.

Lesson Plan: Telling Personal Events

Objective

To use generalized event scripts to structure verbal accounts of personally experienced events.

Materials

Children's books based on familiar generalized event scripts.

Activity

Through conversation or by reading a book out loud, the clinician sets up a context for sharing personal experiences that makes sense. The clinician recounts a personal experience that relates to the context as a demonstration. Students are given the opportunity to tell personal event narratives that are relevant to the context.

Procedure

Demonstration: "You know what? One time I was out walking my three dogs on the street and this big dog came running out from behind his house and tried to attack us! I was so scared that I started screaming and crying at the same time. The big dog went right for my biggest dog Cody's neck. Cody reared up and the two dogs gnashed teeth and growled while my other dogs barked and snarled like crazy! I tried to get the big dog to go away by yelling at it but it just kept trying to bite Cody. Finally the owner of the big dog came running out of his house and shouted a command to his dog. The dog backed off and Cody looked really proud of himself. He sniffed me and my other two dogs over to make sure we were not hurt. After I checked Cody to make sure he wasn't bleeding, I told the owner to keep his dog chained up or I would call the police. The guy didn't even say he was sorry."

- ○ **Clinician:** "Now each of you will have a chance to tell our group about one time when you were really scared. Try to tell what happened in order and remember the scary part because it is the most important thing we want to hear about. "

- ○ **Student:** Each student tells about a personal experience that goes with the topic established by the clinician's demonstration. If a student does not respond, the clinician provides cues.

- ○ **Clinician:** "Let's help you think by making a list of things that are scary." The clinician and the students brainstorm a list.

- ○ **Student:** Each student looks at the list, recalls a personal experience, and tells about it with structurally and content-related support cues provided by the clinician as needed.

Teaching Story Structure: Retelling Episodic Stories

Introduction

Because we know that being able to use a story structure is an excellent predictor of future reading comprehension in young children, it makes sense to focus language intervention for school-aged children on retelling episodic stories. Assuming that they have been read to by their parents or caretakers, typically developing children as young as 4 years of age can retell complete episodes of familiar stories quite easily. Because all children who have been denied opportunities to hear stories struggle with reading comprehension, it stands to reason that children with both limited exposure to stories and language impairment are at great risk for reading failure. We feel strongly that speech-language pathologists can significantly impact academic performance for students with language impairment if they include teaching story structure in their intervention.

Objectives

There are five basic objectives that we use for teaching episodic story structure. The objectives for retelling part of an episode are listed, followed by objectives for retelling complete episodes within a story.

Materials

The most important material needed for story retelling activities of any kind is an episodic story with at least one clear episode. The print text should be covered so that the students cannot view the words. We use as manipulatives three interlocking puzzle pieces to represent the three parts of an episode.

Clinician's Role

The clinician reads aloud an episodic story based on a generalized event script familiar to the students. The story may be either published or clinician constructed. It should be read slowly with both vocal and facial inflection. The clinician must prepare each book that is used in a retelling activity. A master copy of the text is made on a separate sheet of paper and used as a script for the clinician to read aloud. The print text is then covered so that it is not visible to the students as they use the pictures in the book to retell the story.

Next, the clinician activates the students' background knowledge by asking them to tell about any personal experiences that relate to the story. The clinician's role includes creating a context for story retelling, mediating throughout story retelling activities, modeling how to retell stories, and supporting the students as their story retelling abilities improve with practice.

Student's Role

Students listen and attend to the episodic stories read aloud by the speech-language pathologist or teacher. He or she actively participates in retelling parts of episodes at first and then advances to retelling complete episodes. Student use pictures from the book during all retelling activities. The clinician may have students manage the manipulatives as a story retelling is demonstrated to encourage and focus their attention as well as prepare them to use the pictures during future story retelling tasks.

Suggested Cueing Strategies

If the student has difficulty with the retelling any part or all of an episode, we provide verbal cues such as:

- "Tell me about Tom's <u>bike</u> problem."
- "Pippo kept falling off so then Patty tried to fix it by _____."
- "After she put him in the wagon and tied it to the back, Pippo didn't _____."

Note: Try to avoid saying "first he, second he, last he" because that tends to turn the task into a sequencing task and removes the relationship between story parts that is crucial to story comprehension.

Suggested Criteria for Mastery

Once a student demonstrates the ability to tell each part of an episode in a story with one episode independently, we recommend moving on to stories with multiple episodes. Our criteria for mastery of story retelling, is to retell three complete episodes within a story containing at least five episodes. Another indicator of mastery is improved classroom performance in improved reading comprehension.

Lesson Plan: Retelling Parts of an Episode

Objectives

1. To retell "initiating events" within simple episodic stories.
2. To retell "attempts" within simple episodic stories.
3. To retell "consequences" within simple episodic stories.

Materials

- A story with one episode, clear pictures representing each part of the episode, with the text covered from view, and linguistic complexity modified as necessary.

• Manipulatives to retell the story such as a "story puzzle". (We have made puzzle pieces to represent each part of an episode by gluing photocopied pictures from the book to pieces of tag board or fun foam.)

Activity

This activity provides an opportunity for students to hear and retell a story with one episode. Analyzing a story with one episode is a good starting point for intervention, when assessment has indicated the ability to tell personal narratives but an inability to retell any of the episodes in a multiple-episode story. The story is read aloud, retold by the clinician as a demonstration, and then retold by the clinician and a student together. The clinician retells two parts of the episode and the student retells the third, until eventually the student has mastered retelling each part of the episode independently.

Procedure

Demonstration: Mediate for students by explaining that stories have parts that fit together like a puzzle. Tell them that listening to stories and retelling them one part at a time will improve their understanding of the stories they read and hear better than ever. Begin the actual demonstration by introducing the story. Help students bring "world knowledge" to bear by discussing their own personal experiences related to the story. The next step is to read the whole story aloud. Read it slowly, with emphasis on each of the three parts of the episode. Be sure that the students are looking at the pictures in the book as you read.

After reading the whole story, show the story puzzle one piece at a time. In a one episode story, each piece of the puzzle should have a picture from the book that represents one part of the episode. Give each part of the episode a name. (We have called the initiating event the "problem," the attempt to solve the problem the "fix it," and the consequence the "solution.") Demonstrate retelling the story as you fit the three pieces of the puzzle together.

○ **Clinician:** Take apart the pieces of the story puzzle and divide them among the students. Tell them that each one has an important part of the story to retell. Instruct them to retell the story as a group by fitting the parts of the story together while retelling their individual part.

○ **Students:** Each student retells his or her part and puts the pieces of the puzzle together. The first time this activity is undertaken, the children may not arrange the pictures in the correct order (initiating event/attempt/consequence).

○ **Clinician:** Point out that the pieces of the puzzle only fit together if the story is retold so that it makes sense.

○ **Students:** The students retell the story and arrange the puzzle pieces until a logical one-episode story is told.

○ **Clinician:** Once the students have arranged the puzzle pieces correctly, have them practice retelling different parts of the episode. If during assessment a student had particular difficulty retelling one part of an episode more than the others, be sure ample opportunity is provided to practice retelling that part.

Note: Students should be able to see the book at all times during the retelling.

Lesson Plan: Retelling Complete Episodes

Objectives

1. To retell one complete episode within an episodic story.
2. To retell half the episodes within an episodic story.

Materials

- A story with multiple episodes.
- The story should have clear pictures that represent each episode, with print text covered and the story simplified, if necessary.
- Manipulatives to retell the story, such as a story puzzle. (We have made puzzle pieces to represent each part of each episode by gluing photocopied pictures from the book to pieces of tag board or fun foam.)

Activity

This activity provides an opportunity for students to hear and retell stories with multiple episodes. A good starting point for intervention is available if during assessment the student consistently retold one-episode stories. The story is read aloud, retold by the clinician as a demonstration, retold by the clinician and student together, and then eventually independently retold by the student using the pictures.

Procedure

Demonstration: Mediate for students by explaining that stories have parts that fit together like a puzzle and that listening to stories and retelling them one part at a time will help them to understand stories better than ever. Begin the actual demonstration by introducing the story to be sure that the students have brought their "world knowledge" to bear. Then read the whole story aloud. Read it slowly with emphasis on the parts of each episode. Be sure that the students are looking at the pictures as you read.

After reading the whole story, show the "story puzzle" one piece at a time. Each piece of the puzzle should have a picture that represents a part of each episode within the story. Give each part of the episode a name. (We have called the initiating event the "problem," the attempt to solve the problem the "fix it," and the consequence the "solution.") Demonstrate retelling the story as you fit the pieces of the story puzzle together one episode at a time.

- **Clinician:** Take apart the pieces of the story puzzle and divide them up among the students. Tell them that each of them has an important part of the story to retell. Instruct them to retell the story by fitting the parts of the story puzzle together.

- ○ **Students:** Each student retells his or her episode of the story and puts the pieces of the puzzle together. The first time this activity is undertaken, the students may not arrange the pictures in the correct order (initiating event + attempt + consequence).

- ○ **Clinician:** Point out that the pieces of the story puzzle fit only together if the story is retold so that it makes sense.

- ○ **Students:** The students retell the story and arrange the puzzle pieces until all of the episodes are retold.

- ○ **Clinician:** Once the students have arranged the puzzle pieces correctly, have them practice retelling multiple episodes.

Note: Students should be able to see the book at all times during the retelling even if using the manipulatives

Teaching Story Structure: Writing Episodic Stories

Introduction

If it is acknowledged that written language composition is a challenge for students with language impairment, because of the additional processing demands of letter formation, spelling, and a limited capacity to construct and hold in mind the mental models, then strengthening knowledge of narrative structure, in itself, should improve written language performance. However, our direct observation of children with language impairment as they attempt to write stories in their classrooms tells us that we must link story telling directly with story writing one step at a time. Teaching how to apply knowledge of story frameworks to the task of writing original stories has significantly improved the quality of the stories our students compose. In fact, their stories often sound better than those of some of their "typical" peers.

Before you begin to teach strategies for improving written language performance, be sure to review the written language curriculum your school is using. Our methodology fits with the underlying principles of process writing. In other words, the two lessons in this section center on using a story map, which is considered a "prewriting" tool. There are several types of graphic organizers presented in students' language arts texts and the literature on teaching written language skills. We use a story map outline that is linear, simple, and easy to reconstruct, so that, eventually, students can visualize it during prewriting activities.

We also recommend focusing strictly on strategies for developing story content during these lessons. They are part of the "planning" and "drafting" phases of the writing process. Later, as students take their story through the remainder of the writing process, spelling, grammar, punctuation, and handwriting can be addressed.

Objectives

Our objectives for writing episodic stories correlate with the writing process as outlined in many language arts curriculums. They focus on teaching students strategies for planning and drafting episodic stories. The first six objectives deal with composing story extensions. Those that follow refer to composition of original stories.

Materials

When planning and drafting a story extension, a familiar episodic story is needed to "add on to." A student either plans and drafts another episode to extend an existing story or replaces an episode in an existing story to change the plot. In both activities, students use a story map outline to guide their planning and drafting. When planning and drafting an original story, all that is needed is a story starter (an idea) and a story map outline.

Clinician's Role

The clinician's role is to create opportunities for students to use their world knowledge and apply their understanding of story structure to produce written narratives. The clinician models how to extend existing stories and compose original stories using a story map outline to plan episodes. The clinician also supports students as they transform ideas from an outline into written sentences that tell a logical, coherent story.

Student's Role

The student either extends an existing story or writes an original one by completing a story map outline during the planning phase of the writing process. After that, the student uses the plan to draft sentences that extend or tell an episodic story.

Suggested Cueing Strategies

By the time students are ready for writing episodes to extend or compose episodic stories, they are familiar with the names that have been assigned to each part of an episode. These names are used to cue students as they complete the planning and drafting of their episodes. For example, "Don't forget to include a way to 'fix' the 'problem' in this part of your story." Or, "Let's brainstorm some other ways to 'fix' the 'bike problem' in your story. The 'solution' you have written doesn't quite make sense."

During drafting activities, students often need support transforming ideas written on the story map outline into sentences that clearly communicate their episode(s). They often copy the information from their story map onto a clean sheet of paper without adding the cohesive devices that make the story stick together. The clinician provides cues that help the story sound like a narrative as students go from the episode planning stage to the episode drafting stage.

Suggested Criteria for Mastery

Remember that the goal is to provide students with strategies for applying the narrative skills they have acquired to the written language task of writing. We have found that a student who can independently "map out" an episode that extends a story using a story map outline is ready to plan and draft an original story with two or three episodes. A student who independently plans and drafts multiple episodes that clearly relate a story has mastered the initial stages of the writing process and is ready to focus on editing for spelling, grammar, punctuation, and letter formation.

Lesson Plan: Writing Episodes to Extend a Story

Objectives

1. To plan an episode that extends a story, given 2 out of 3 parts.
2. To plan an episode that extends a story, given 1 out of 3 parts.
3. To plan 1 complete episode that extends a story.
4. To plan 2 complete episodes that extend a story.
5. To draft an episode that extends a story, given 2 out of 3 parts.
6. To draft an episode that extends a story, given 1 out of 3 parts.
7. To draft 1 complete episode that extends a story.
8. To draft 2 complete episodes that extend a story.

Materials

- An episodic story with clear pictures and text covered, with story modified as needed.
- A story map outline with 2 parts filled in.

   Example:

   The boy wanted to play in the snow but he couldn't find his mittens. (IE)

   He looked all around and then he asked his mother. (A)

   _____ (C)

Activity

The clinician reads an episodic story aloud. The students listen to the story and look at the pictures. The clinician and students brainstorm ideas for extending the story by adding an episode or changing the story by replacing an episode. Students are given a one-episode story map with two parts filled in to use as a graphic organizer. Gradually they learn to fill in each part of an episode that extends a story with no support from the clinician.

Procedures

Demonstration: Mediate for the students. Explain to them that, "Students are often asked to write their own stories in school. We can begin by writing new parts (episodes) to stories that we are reading."

○ **Clinician:** Read the whole story aloud. Be sure that the students are looking at the pictures.

○ **Students:** Retell the story aloud as a group.

○ **Clinician:** Discuss the plot of the story as you take apart each episode using a story map outline. At the end of the story, plan a new episode that keeps the story going or changes the way the story ends. Provide students with a story map that has two parts of the new episode filled in. Help students brainstorm ways to complete the plan for the new episode.

○ **Students:** Students select an idea for completing the plan for the new episode and write it on the story map outline. Students then retell the episode to be sure it makes sense.

○ **Clinician:** The clinician writes a draft of the new episode as the students retell it using the story map as a guide. The clinician reads the whole story aloud, including the new episode.

○ **Students:** The students gradually take over the task of planning and drafting the new episode using a story map outline.

Lesson Plan: Writing Original Episodic Stories
(A Small Group Lesson)

Objectives

1. To plan an original episode, given 2 out of 3 parts.
2. To plan an original episode, given 1 out of 3 parts.
3. To plan 1 original episode.
4. To plan 2 original episodes.
5. To draft an original episode, given 2 out of 3 parts.
6. To draft an original episode, given 1 out of 3 parts.
7. To draft 1 original episode.
8. To draft 2 original episodes.

Materials

- An episodic story with clear pictures and text covered, with story modified as needed.
- A story map outline with 2 parts filled-in.

Activity

The clinician and the students brainstorm ideas for an original story. Students are encouraged to draw from personal experiences, based on generalized event scripts. The clinician and the students use a story map as a graphic organizer to plan and draft an original story containing at least two complete episodes.

Procedures

Demonstration: Mediate for the students by saying, "Students are often asked to write their own stories in school. Now that we can add to or change stories that someone else has written, we are ready to turn our own ideas into stories and write them down for others to read." Model for students how to brainstorm a list of personal experiences to write about, or how to select a story starter from a list provided by the classroom teacher. Fill in a story map outline with at least two episodes. Think out loud as you suggest characters and the setting. Continue to verbalize your thought process as you develop a "problem," a way to "fix it," and a "solution" followed by another "problem," a way to "fix it," and a "solution." Record all of your ideas on the story map outline and retell the story aloud using it as a guide. Finally, model how to take information from the outline and turn it into written sentences that tell a story.

- ○ **Clinician:** Write students' ideas for stories based on personal experiences on the chalkboard or dry erase board.

- ○ **Students:** Choose an idea for an individual story or decide as a group to select an idea and write a story together.

- ○ **Clinician:** Coach students as they brainstorm characters, a setting, and an initiating event (problem) for the first episode in the story.

- ○ **Students:** Choose characters and the setting. Select an initiating event for the first episode in the story.

- ○ **Clinician:** Coach students as they brainstorm attempts to solve the problem (fix its) in the first episode of the story.

- ○ **Students:** Choose an attempt (fix it) for the first episode in the story.

- ○ **Clinician:** Coach students as they brainstorm possible consequences for the first episode in the story.

- ○ **Students:** Retell the first episode to make sure the three parts of the episode fit together and make sense.

- ○ **Clinician:** Repeat this process for the second episode. Keep students focused on the concept that the parts of each episode must fit together and that the episodes themselves must tell a story that makes sense.

Lesson Plan: Teaching Carryover of Written Narrative Skills (This lesson can be completed in cooperative groups or individually)

Objectives

1. To plan 2 original episodes.
2. To draft 2 original episodes.

Materials

- • Examples of episodic stories. A "series" with several different titles such as *Curious George*, *Billy and Blaze*, and *Nate the Great Books*.

- Partially completed story map outlines for each student or cooperative group in the classroom
- Blank story map outlines for each student or cooperative group in the classroom

Activity

The purpose of this activity is to provide an opportunity for **all** students to plan and draft an episodic story of their own to the best of their ability. Some students will need minimal support to write stories with four or five episodes; others will require significant support to write one with two episodes. Another few students, even with maximum support, will struggle with simply completing the story map outline.

This lesson is recommended for students in at least third grade. It is to be presented by the speech-language pathologist along with a classroom teacher and/or a special education teacher. Before participating in this carryover activity, students with language impairment should have completed lessons for planning and drafting story extensions and original stories. The clinician and teacher(s) will coach all students throughout the activity, as needed.

Procedures

Demonstration: Mediate for the students. Introduce the concept of an episodic story using a story with one or two episodes. Use the terms "problem," "fix it," and "solution" and take the story apart one episode at a time. Record the parts of the episode(s) on a story map outline. When students seem to understand the concept of an "episode" and how to take it apart, continue with the lesson. The students with language impairment should be familiar with these concepts already, because of their prior experience with planning and drafting episodic stories.

- ○ **Clinician/Teacher:** Read aloud one episodic story from a series. Show a completed story map for the story on an overhead projector or computerized projection. Review the process of "taking the story apart" and label the parts of the episode.

- ○ **Teacher:** Divide the class into small groups. Have each group read an episodic story from the selected series. Give each group a partially completed story map for their story. Have group members fill in the missing parts of the episodes on the story map. Have each group retell their story aloud using their completed story map as a guide.

- ○ **Clinician/Teacher:** Have the whole class brainstorm ideas for adding another story to the series. (e.g., Write a new *Billy and Blaze* adventure.) Record all ideas for new stories so that the students can refer to the list when it comes time for them to plan their stories.

- ○ **Teacher:** Divide the class into cooperative groups. Instruct each group to plan an original episodic story using a story map outline.

- ○ **Teacher:** Have each group tell their story aloud to an adult in the classroom to be sure it fits an episodic framework before they begin to draft their story. Through mediation, help students modify their story maps so that they clearly outline two episodes.

○ **Teacher:** Have students individually draft an episodic story using the outline. Continue to take the story through the writing process until it is a finished product. Provide opportunities to illustrate each episode of their stories and share them with others.

APPENDIX 6A

Story Map Outline

Title: _____

Author: _____

Setting: _____

Main Characters: _____

Episode #1

Important Event/Problem: _____

_____

Attempt to deal with/solve it: _____

_____

Consequence/Solution: _____

_____

Episode #2

Important Event/Problem: _____

_____

Attempt to deal with/solve it: _____

_____

Consequence/Solution: _____

_____

PART III
Advanced Literacy Skills

CHAPTER

7

Introduction to Advanced Literacy Skills

> Readers who see the trees and not the forest have difficulty in connecting information across the text and often get "lost" in what they read without any recognition that they do not understand. More global readers tend to stick with an early, vague idea and not change it, even when a good many ideas do not support their initial impression.
>
> Blachowicz (1994), p. 307

The description of two avenues to reading failure given by Blachowicz (1994) captures the problems many children with language impairments have when they attempt to comprehend what they read. Either they focus on details, often trivial details, in a text without regard to the meaning or structure of the whole text, or they focus on an idea about what the text might be saying, perhaps gleaned from a chapter title or heading and ignore details that might extend or clarify the meaning of the text. These difficulties with reading comprehension are magnified when a child with a language impairment tries to write an original composition, whether an essay or a story. Any sense of how to communicate a main idea, how to marshal supporting details, and how to organize the text appears to be either absent or unavailable to the child (Westby, 1998).

Why should *SLPs* assess and train a child's ability to use advanced literacy skills?

The word "SLPs" is emphasized in the question, because many school speech-language pathologists avoid working in this area of language use at all. There are probably several reasons for this, but the two most apparent are:

- It's the teacher's job, not mine. I don't teach reading and writing.
- I don't know enough about what the child needs to know to be able to work in this area.

To both of these statements, we respond with the following reasoning:

- It is the job of the school speech-language pathologist to foster and support the academic learning of the children in her or his caseload. If our work is not relevant to the child's academic progress, then it is not relevant to the child's most important needs.
- We can train the child with a language impairment to develop metacognitive strategies that will assist in reading comprehension and in writing assignments. These may be the same strategies being taught in the child's classroom, and our reason for working with them is simple: Children with language impairments need slower presentation and more repetition of new information. They also need many more opportunities to practice using a newly learned strategy than the typical classroom can provide. Providing this repetition and opportunity for practice is our job. The short answer to the question is, because we owe it to the children on our caseloads.

What are the classroom implications of training a child's ability to use strategies to improve advanced literacy skills?

Students who have difficulty comprehending what they read or who struggle to compose a text more than three sentences long are often the same children who are classified as having "communication impairment" or "learning disabilities." As these students progress through the later elementary grades into middle school and high school, they tend to fall farther and farther behind academically. This is not so much because they lack the ability to understand the content of the curriculum as because they lack access to this content because of their poor reading comprehension. Then, even when they are able to comprehend, they have difficulty demonstrating their comprehension or applying their knowledge to solve problems, because their writing skills are so poor that it's hard to know exactly what they know. Any work SLPs do that improves this situation for these children will have a positive impact on their academic performance.

What evidence is there that training of this sort works? Direct strategy instruction as a way of teaching children to identify main ideas has been evaluated by Baumann (1984a, 1986b) and by Williams (1984). Taylor and Williams (1983) compared the effectiveness of such intervention for fourth and fifth grade children with learning disabilities versus normally achieving children matched for word knowledge. The researchers' results make it clear that instruction designed to develop main idea skills should not necessarily be different for children with learning disabilities than for other children. Williams and her colleagues (1983) also conducted a study to determine whether improvements in main idea skills shown by the children in their study were due to the intervention they did or to general classroom instruction. They found that the group receiving instruction performed significantly better on a test of main idea identification than a comparison group of children from the same classrooms. These results confirm those of Baumann (1986b) concerning the effectiveness of a direct instruction paradigm with sixth grade students. Direct strategy instruction also seems to work when teaching children to make inferences to connect information across a text (Hansen & Pearson, 1983; Raphael, 1982). Children can be taught to integrate information in the text with their prior knowledge (Sentell & Blachowicz, 1989).

In this section, we present:

- Assessment techniques for use in determining a child's level of ability with main idea and inferencing, together with information about how to interpret the results obtained from such assessments.
- Examples of goals and objectives useful when writing about main idea and inferencing abilities on a child's IEP.
- Examples of lesson plans illustrating techniques for instructing children about strategies to be used for detecting main ideas and for inferencing.

CHAPTER

8

Assessment of Advanced Literacy Skills

Finding the Main Idea

Finding the main idea of a text is a complex task, involving a child's knowledge of language and text conventions on many levels. It is important for children as they move through the later grades of elementary school because so many of the tasks they will be called on to do depend on finding a main idea. A child who cannot determine the main idea of a text has difficulty answering the apparently simple question, "What is this text about?" Imagine being asked to outline a chapter in a book or to write a summary for a unit of text without being able to decide what the chapter or the unit might be about! Most, if not all, children with language impairments struggle with assignments of this sort. Their difficulties may arise because they have not mastered underlying skills (such as pronoun reference or, perhaps, inferencing abilities). They also may lack strategies for attempting to deal with a body of text as a whole unit, and their attempt to do this stresses their language processing ability beyond their ability to perform.

Baumann (1986) presents a sequence of main idea tasks organized in terms of the grade level at which a child should be able to do each one. This sequence, presented next, forms the basis for our assessment task.

Sequence of Main Idea Tasks

Find main idea in lists of words	Grade 1
Find main idea in sentences	Grade 2
Find main idea and details in paragraphs where main idea is explicitly stated or	Grade 3
where main idea is implicitly stated	later Grade 3
Find main ideas and details in short passages (more than one paragraph) where main idea is explicitly stated or where main idea is	Grade 5
implicitly stated	later Grade 5
Compose main idea outlines	Grade 6
Find main idea in long passages (such as a textbook chapter)	Grade 7

The Main Idea Task

> Comprehension of main idea rests strongly on basic categorization and classification skills.
>
> Baumann (1986), p. 94

This task is designed to be used as a way to determine the level at which a child can identify what is common to a set of pictures, words, phrases, or sentences. It is designed to increase the level of language processing a child must engage in at each level. It is based on Baumann's (1984) assertion that main idea comprehension is an extension of basic categorization and classification skills. A child who can identify what a set of pictures has in common and choose another picture that belongs to that set is demonstrating basic categorization and classification skills. A child who can read a paragraph and then pick from a set of three sentences the one that would fit in the paragraph is demonstrating not only basic categorization and classification skills, but also the ability to apply these skills to text. The main idea assessment instrument is not intended to diagnose a language impairment, but rather to provide information about where to begin classroom-relevant intervention with a child already so identified. We do not advise using this assessment task for children with language impairments who are not at least in third grade, primarily because we doubt that much would be learned from it before that time. Most of our use of this instrument has involved children in grade 3 or above who have been labeled as having communication impairment or a learning disability. We have not found any children at grade 3 or above who could not respond correctly to the picture items or to the lists of single words. The assessment task begins with pictures only for one reason: If a child cannot read and has an auditory memory problem causing the student to be unable to process text that is read to him or her, starting at the picture level will at least tell us something about the child's basic ability to categorize. We begin to see variations in performance as we move to sentences and paragraphs, where some children can still perform accurately and others begin to fail.

The assessment instrument consists of sets of pictures, single words, phrases, sentences, and sentences organized into short paragraphs. In each instance, a child views a set of three pictures, words, and so on (the target set) and is then asked to view a second set of three (the alternative set) and tell which single item from the second set belongs with the first set. For example, the child might see a set of three target pictures: a pair of gloves, a scarf, and a jacket. Then the child looks at a second set of alternative pictures: a fireman, a sled, and a knitted cap, and is asked to tell which picture from the alternative set belongs with the target set. Whether the child is looking at pictures, words, sentences, or paragraphs, the response consists entirely of pointing and no expressive language is demanded from the child. The assumption behind this procedure is that a child must be able to decide what the target set has in common (the main idea) to choose the appropriate answer from the alternative set. When we used this task, we mounted each set of target items onto a 5" × 7" index card, and each set of alternative items on another card, with the alternatives clearly separated from each other. We then put each card into a clear plastic page in a looseleaf notebook so that the child could see the target set and the set of alternatives at the same time. Whether you decide to do this, or simply to use the cards without putting them into a notebook, it is important that the child be able to see the target items and the alternative items **at the same time.** This is not a memory task and we want to give all the visual support possible.

Administration

Directions

The directions are intended to familiarize the child with the task. The directions are written, with feedback, provided for correct responses. If the child gives incorrect responses to the trial items presented in the directions, simply correct the child's response by saying "Look again. The ____ goes with these three pictures (or words, or sentences, etc.)." It is best to go through the entire set of directions and trial items, and then begin the test. Provide feedback only for the trial items. Once the test items begin, do not provide feedback about correct answers, but only about how hard the child is working.

Before you begin administering the test items, it will be important to be sure that your cards are in the correct order. Otherwise, it will be extremely difficult for you to mark the score sheet as the child responds. For each item on the test, the correct answer is presented in bold type on the score sheet. You need only indicate which item the child pointed to. At the conclusion of the task, attend to the level at which the child began to give numerous incorrect responses (words, sentences, etc.) It is at that level that intervention should probably begin.

Interpreting Responses

It is a good idea to get additional information about why a child is giving incorrect answers for a set of items. To get this information, you may want to ask the child to explain why she or he pointed to a particular item. It will probably be advisable to do this not only for items the child misses, but also for items the child gets correctly. Sometimes this will reveal errors the child has made in interpreting the items, and sometimes it will reveal the child's inability to extract from the stimulus items the critical information related to classification. For example:

Stimulus paragraph: *Grandmother's house is full of nice furniture. Tony fell asleep on grandmother's bed. We sat on grandmother's couch to watch TV. Liz did her homework at grandmother's desk.*

Alternative sentences:

1. *Mary spilled milk on grandmother's rug.*
2. *Grandmother's coffeepot is empty.*
3. *We had lunch at grandmother's kitchen table.*

One child chose item #1 to go with the stimulus paragraph. When asked why he chose it, he said that the paragraph was about furniture, and a rug was a kind of furniture. We would not consider this an indication that the child could not find the underlying idea in a paragraph. It might be an indication that he doesn't know how to classify rugs, but surely this is a trivial error. A more serious error would be revealed by a child who chose item #1 and reported that she did so because Mary always goes to her grandmother's house. This sort of error indicates a failure on the child's part to understand what the paragraph is about or how to relate new information to an underlying topic.

If you choose to ask a child why particular responses were chosen, you may want to write the child's answers on the answer sheet for your future reference.

Using the task to decide who needs intervention

As with other tasks in this book, you may wish to establish your own local norms or average standards, simply to give you some idea about what level of performance a teacher might be expecting from the average child in a particular grade in your school system. It is useful to administer this task to four or five average children from the same classroom as your target child. This not only gives you a sense for what "average" children can do, but also provides you with information to use when you talk with parents or teachers about the problems of a child with language impairment or learning disability. Having scores from average children enables you to say something like, "the score on this task for average children in your child's classroom is between X and Y. Your child scored Z. As you can see, his performance is well below what we might expect from an average achiever. This indicates that your child might profit from some training in how to find the main idea of text that he reads."

Inferencing Assessment

> Reading comprehension failure can arise from children's difficulties in integrating information within a story and using general knowledge to deduce what is not explicitly stated.
>
> Bishop and Adams (1990), p. 127

In using prior experience and knowledge of the world to interpret what is read, individuals engage in constructive comprehension or inferencing. This activity is common to all skilled readers, and often occurs without the reader even being aware of it. For example, consider the following passage, used to introduce a novel:

> *Marian walked slowly through the sand, thinking about what she would do when Jake arrived. She felt the warm water lapping around her ankles, and realized that she should get back to the house before the water cut off her passage around the rocks. She wondered when high tide would be.*

We realize, without being explicitly told, that Marian is on a beach beside the ocean. We also realize that there is some sort of problem connected with Jake's arrival, although this was not explicitly stated either. This sort of constructive comprehension allows readers to begin to establish a framework, or a context, within which the text that follows will be interpreted. As we continued to read, the construction of this context both guides interpretations of the text and is affected by further details.

Research (Bishop & Adams, 1990; Crais & Chapman, 1987; Ellis Weismer, 1985) suggests that children with language impairments have great difficulty with inferencing, or constructive comprehension. The general finding is that their performance is like that of normally developing children who are 2 to 3 years younger. There are several possible reasons why children with language impairments fail to make inferences as they read. In some cases, they may simply lack sufficient world knowledge to adequately interpret the text they are confronted with, because they either have limited experience or fail to store or retrieve memories of that experience. They also may not be able to apply their memories of their experience in relevant situations because of processing limitations. A child must be able to use textual cues to call up relevant information from memory (for example, *sand, water, tide* in the passage above). Then selected bits of that information must be used to construct a framework or context that is held in the mind and, perhaps, amended as further text is encountered. A child with language impairment may fail to see the important textual cues, may be unable to choose the most relevant parts of stored information, or may be unable to hold on to the context constructed as the child gets further into the text and has to interpret complex language.

A Task for Assessing Inferencing Abilities

The key points to remember when attempting to discover if a child is able to make appropriate inferences about a text are:

- Be certain that the child has relevant world knowledge to apply to the task. This means that SLPs must ascertain in advance if a child has had experience (direct or vicarious) with the events or situations covered in the text.
- Be certain that the text itself is within the child's comprehension level. A sixth grader whose reading ability is at a third grade level will not be likely to apply constructive comprehension skills to a sixth grade text. This is simply because the demands associated with unfamiliar vocabulary words and more complex sentences will overwhelm the student. Third grade level text will be more likely to eliminate vocabulary or word recognition difficulties.

With this in mind, we have constructed a set of brief scenarios, together with questions to use in determining if a child makes inferences when confronted with a text. If your knowledge of a given child's experience suggests that the situations covered in these scenarios will be unfamiliar to the child, you might try constructing your own scenarios to fit with what the child knows, or you might just use the ones from this set that seem appropriate.

Administration

Directions

You will need to have a copy of the scenarios (without the questions on it) to put in front of the child and a copy with the questions on it to use as a score sheet. Say to the child, "I am going to read some little stories to you, and then I'll ask you some questions about each story. You will have the stories in front of you, so you can read along with me."

After reading the text to the child, ask the questions you have prepared. The text remains in front of the child at all times, so that this does not become a memory task.

Interpreting Responses

This is another of those tasks that necessitate knowing what the average achiever in the target child's classroom is capable of doing. In this case, the SLP should probably ask the teacher for the names of four or five children whose reading comprehension is at grade level, and then go through this task with them to get a sense of how they perform. The SLP would then have some basis for judging whether the target child needs work with inferencing. Such information would also make it easier to talk with parents, teachers, and others about why inferencing was being included in the child's IEP. Be able to say that "average readers in this child's classroom are able to respond correctly to X number of these items, but the target child was able to respond only to Y number. This suggests that the child needs practice with constructive comprehension skills to facilitate his reading comprehension."

How to talk about advanced literacy skills at the IEP conference

Often, SLPs need to remind teachers and parents that children with language impairment have particular difficulty comprehending the material in their textbooks, because their poor vocabularies and their difficulties with decoding add to their processing loads as they try to read. This means they will need extra help as they work toward grade-level reading comprehension.

It is important to be able to explain to teachers and parents alike that you are not attempting to "take over" what the teacher does in the classroom. You are simply providing opportunities for children with language impairment to get more practice in language use by having repeated instruction with these abilities. It will also be important to explain that you will be training *strategies* for the child to use as the student encounters the content in the classroom and that you will not teach that content.

When talking about specific assessment results, the kind of informal comparisons we have advocated throughout this book should be sufficient. That is, to say "the average reader in your child's classroom can correctly complete X of these items, and your child completed Y." We need to emphasize that this is informal, criterion- based assessment conducted primarily to find out where work with the child should be targeted.

APPENDIX 8A

The Inferencing Assessment Task

1. Katie and Josh carried presents in their hands as they came into the room. They were looking forward to eating cake and singing while Matt blew out the candles.

    Questions:

    A. What did Katie and Josh carry in their hands?

    B. Where were Katie and Josh going?

    C. Who were the presents for?

2. Josh went up to the counter and ordered his food. His mother took money out of her purse and looked around for a place to sit. The man behind the counter put the food on a tray and gave it to Josh.

    Questions:

    A. What kind of food do you think Josh might have ordered?

    B. Why did Josh's mom take money out of her purse?

    C. What did the man behind the counter do with the food?

3. Katie raised her hand and said, "I need to sharpen my pencil." The teacher told her to hurry, because they would soon be going to lunch. Katie sharpened her pencil and put it in her desk before she got in line.

    Questions:

    A. Why did Katie get in line?

    B. Why did the teacher tell her to hurry?

    C. Where was Katie when she asked to sharpen her pencil?

4. Katie threw the ball as Josh stood at the plate. He tried to hit the ball, but he missed. Katie said, "that's strike one." Josh said, "I'll hit the next one."

    Questions:

    A. What game are Katie and Josh playing?

    B. What did Josh have in his hands when he tried to hit the ball?

    C. What did Katie say when Josh missed the ball?

4. Josh heard the bell ring as he got off the bus. He hurried through the hall to get to his classroom. He did not like being late.

    Questions:

    A. How did Josh get to school?

    B. Where was Josh hurrying to go?

    C. Why did Josh not like being late?

6. Katie put on her pajamas and brushed her teeth. Her mother tucked her in and said goodnight. Katie said, "will you leave the light on?"

   Questions:

   A. Why did Katie ask her mother to leave the light on?

   B. Where was Katie when she asked her mother to leave the light on?

   C. What did Katie put on?

7. Josh sat on the table while the nurse looked in his ears. He said, "my throat is sore." The nurse asked him to open his mouth and say "ahhh."

   Questions:

   A. Where is Josh?

   B. Why is Josh at the doctor's office?

   C. What did the nurse ask Josh to do?

8. Josh and Katie helped to decorate the tree. Josh brought a string of lights to put on it and Katie had a star to put on top. When they finished, they went outside to make a snowman.

   Questions:

   A. What holiday are Josh and Katie getting ready for?

   B. What did Josh bring to put on the tree?

   C. What season of the year is it?

Inference Assessment Score Sheet

Instructions: Read the paragraph to the child as the student follows along on his or her copy. Read the questions to the child one at a time and write down answers. Mark the answer correct (+) or incorrect (−) based on what other children in his classroom or at his reading level did on this question.

Paragraph 1   +/−

Question A: _____   ____

_____

Question B: _____   ____

_____

Question C: _____   ____

_____

Paragraph 2

Question A: _____   ____

_____

Question B: _____   ____

_____

Question C: _____   ____

_____

Paragraph 3

Question A: _____   ____

_____

Question B: _____   ____

_____

Question C: _____   ____

_____

Paragraph 4   +/−

Question A: _____   ____

_____

Question B: _____   ____

_____

Question C: _____   ____

_____

Paragraph 5

Question A: _____   ____

_____

Question B: _____   ____

_____

Question C: _____   ____

_____

Paragraph 6

Question A: _____   ____

_____

Question B: _____   ____

_____

Question C: _____   ____

_____

Paragraph 7

Question A: _____   ____

_____

+/−

Question B: _____   _____

_____

Question C: _____   _____

_____

Paragraph 8

Question A: _____   _____

_____

Question B: _____   _____

_____

Question C: _____   _____

_____

APPENDIX 8B

The Main Idea Task

Directions

1. Today, we're going to do some work on figuring out **main ideas**. Main idea is not a hard thing to figure out. Let me give you an example. I have some pictures here. You know what these pictures are, I'll bet. Look at these and tell me what they are. (Point to Example target pictures, one at a time, allow child to label them.)

   Here are some other pictures. Look at these and tell me what they are. (Point to Example alternative pictures one at a time and allow child to label them.)

   One of these pictures (point to set of alternative pictures) goes with this group of pictures (point to target set.) Which of these pictures goes with this group of pictures?

   Right. The picture of the grapes goes with these pictures. (Point to correct picture together with target set.) You were able to pick out the right picture because you knew the main idea that makes all these pictures go together. They are all fruit and you knew that grapes are also fruit.

2. Now let's try this with some words. Can you read the words in this group? (Allow child to read the words in the Example target set. Provide help if necessary.) Now here are three more words. Can you read these words? (Point to Example alternative set, one at a time. Provide help if necessary.) One of these words (point to alternative choices) goes with the words in this group (point to target group). Can you tell me which word it is?

   Right. The word "train" goes with these words, because they are all things we ride in, or kinds of transportation.

3. Now let's try some phrases, or two words together. Can you read the phrases on this list? (Allow child to read the phrases in the Example target set. Provide help if necessary.) Now here are three more words. Can you read these words? (Point to Example alternative choices. Aid in decoding if necessary.) One of these phrases (point to alternative choices) goes with the phrases in this group (point to target group). Which of these phrases goes with this group of phrases?

   Right. The phrase "fast deer" goes with this group, because they are all about animals.

4. Now we'll try some sentences. Let's read the sentences on this page. (Allow child to read sentences in the Example target set. Provide help if necessary.) Now here are three more sentences. Let's read these sentences. (Point to Example alternative choices. Provide help if necessary.)

Which one of these sentences (point to alternative set) goes with these (point to target set)? Yes, the sentence "Mary's doll is pretty" is the right choice, because all these sentences are about toys.

5. The last thing we'll work on is paragraphs. Let's read this paragraph (point to Example target paragraph. Provide reading help if needed.) One of these sentences here (point to Example alternative set) belongs in this paragraph. Let's read the sentences and see if you can tell which one belongs in the paragraph. (Point to alternative sentences one at a time. Provide reading help if needed.) Which one do you think belongs in the paragraph? The sentence about grapes belongs, doesn't it? It belongs because this is a paragraph about fruit and grapes are a kind of fruit.

6. OK. We've had a chance to practice these. Now we'll do some others. They will be exactly like the ones we just did. I will show you some pictures, or words, or phrases, or sentences, and you will decide which ones belong together. Ready? Here's the first one.

Proceed with test items

Scoring Sheet for Main Idea Task

Date _____

Name _____ Age _____ Grade _____

1.	a	b	**c**	10.	**a**	b	c	19.	a	**b**	c
2.	a	b	**c**	11.	**a**	b	c	20.	a	b	**c**
3.	a	**b**	c	12.	a	**b**	c	21.	a	**b**	c
4.	a	**b**	c	13.	**a**	b	c	22.	a	b	**c**
5.	**a**	b	c	14.	**a**	b	c	23.	a	b	**c**
6.	**a**	b	c	15.	**a**	b	c	24.	a	b	**c**
7.	a	b	**c**	16.	a	b	**c**	25.	**a**	b	c
8.	**a**	b	c	17.	a	**b**	c				
9.	a	b	**c**	18.	**a**	b	c				

EXAMPLE

1 Target Set

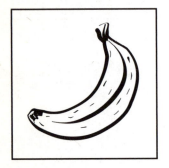 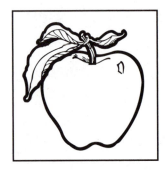 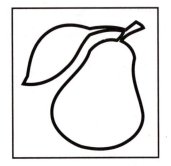

Alternatives

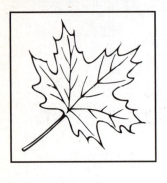 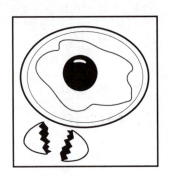 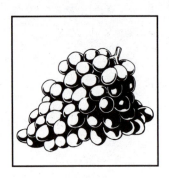

A   B   C

EXAMPLE

2 Target Set

Car

Truck

Airplane

Alternatives

Train   **House**   **Gas station**

A   **B**   **C**

EXAMPLE

3 Target Set

Red fox

Wise owl

Fat squirrel

Alternatives

Green bush   **Fast deer**   **Big grasshopper**

A   **B**   **C**

EXAMPLE

4 Target Set

Balls can bounce on the sidewalk.

Kites fly high in the sky.

Bikes need to have good brakes.

Alternatives

A   Dolls can wear pretty clothes.

B   Some boys are quite tall.

C   Flags wave in the wind

EXAMPLE

5 Target Set

Fruit is very good for us. Many children like bananas. My mom likes the taste of apples. Courtney eats pears for lunch.

Alternatives

A   We had grapes for a snack.

B   Dad eats fried eggs for breakfast.

C   Birds like to eat worms.

Main Idea Test Items

1. Target Set

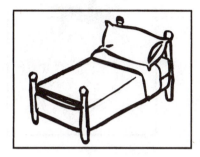 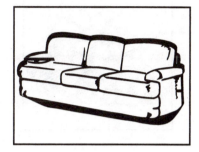 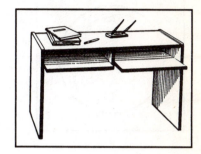

Alternatives

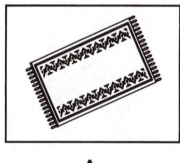 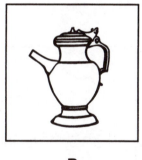 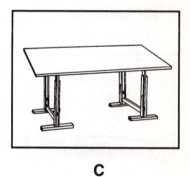

A	B	C

2. Target Set

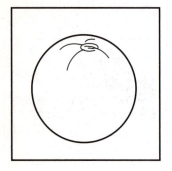
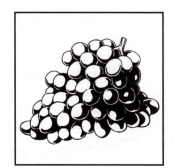
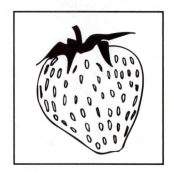

Alternatives

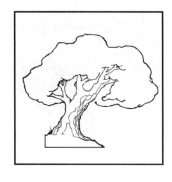
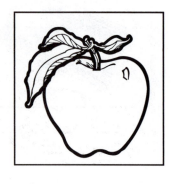

A   B   C

3. Target Set

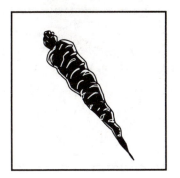 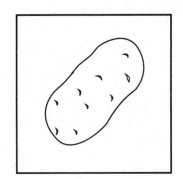 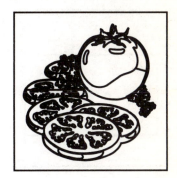

Alternatives

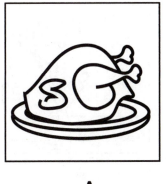 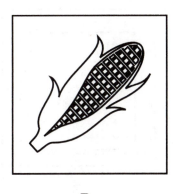 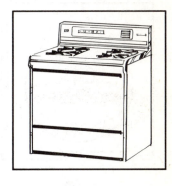

A  B C

4. Target Set

 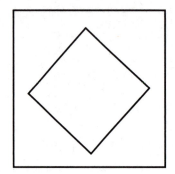 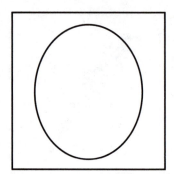

Alternatives

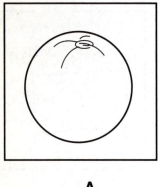  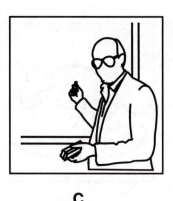

A   **B**   **C**

5. Target Set

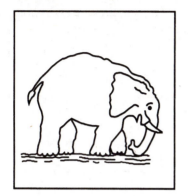 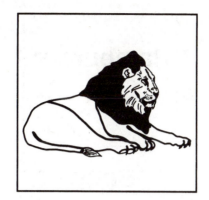 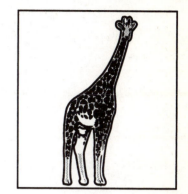

Alternatives

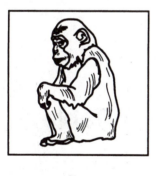  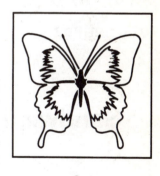

A   **B**   **C**

6. Target Set

Hamburger

Soup

Pizza

Alternatives

Sandwich   **Man**   **Table**

A   B   C

7. Target Set

Train

Ship

Bus

Alternatives

Fireman   **Lawnmower**   **Truck**

A   B   C

8. Target Set

Cow

Pig

Rooster

Alternatives

Lamb   Snake   Corn

A   B   C

9. Target Set

School

Church

House

Alternatives

Van   Fence   Barn

A   **B**   **C**

10. Target Set

Tree

Flower

Vine

Alternatives

Bush   **Saw**   **Vase**

A   **B**   **C**

11. Target Set

Brave fireman

Smart teacher

Kind nurse

Alternatives

Busy mailman   **Warm hat**   **Yellow bus**

A   **B**   **C**

12. Target Set

Black dog

Furry cat

Fast horse

Alternatives

Long fence   **Big elephant**   **Colorful bird**

A   B   C

13. Target Set

Spotted cow

Dirty pig

Loud rooster

Alternatives

Soft lamb	Long snake	Yellow corn
A	**B**	**C**

14. Target Set

Small circle

Yellow square

Big triangle

Alternatives

Long rectangle   Full jar   Red crayon

A   B   C

15. Target Set

Pretty sister

Strong dad

Old grandmother

Alternatives

Little brother	Furry cat	Big house
A	**B**	**C**

16. Target Set

Shirts can be too big.

Dresses are sometimes pink.

Jeans are always blue.

Alternatives

A   The girl is too young.

B   The church is very quiet.

C   Her skirt is striped.

17. Target Set

Bears can be black.

Monkeys act so silly.

Kangaroos like to hop.

Alternatives

A   Knives are sometimes sharp.

B   Lions are very fierce.

C   Trees have green leaves.

18. Target Set

Balloons can be red.

Dolls are often pretty.

Footballs have white laces.

Alternatives

A   **Bikes are fun to ride.**

B   **Monkeys like to eat peanuts.**

C   **Dad drives a new car.**

19. Target Set

Turtles walk very slowly

Crocodiles live in rivers.

Snakes crawl on the ground.

Alternatives

A   Butterflies like the flowers.

B   Lizards are usually small.

C   Jungles might be scary.

20. Target Set

Grasshoppers live in the grass.

Flies make buzzing noises.

Butterflies have beautiful wings.

Alternatives

A   Snakes are not slimy.

B   Plants like lots of water.

C   Moths fly around the lamp.

21. Target Set

Vegetables are full of vitamins. Rabbits like to nibble on carrots. Paula's favorite food is mashed potatoes. Kim puts tomato on her sandwich.

Alternatives

A   We had roast turkey for Thanksgiving.

B   Everyone likes to eat corn on the cob.

C   Don't touch the hot stove.

22.Target Set

Fruit makes a good snack after school. Andy peeled his orange before he ate it. Betty ate her grapes one at a time. Charlie ate every one of his strawberries.

Alternatives

A   We had chicken soup for lunch.

B   A big limb fell off the tree.

C   Jennifer ate an apple yesterday.

23. Target Set

Lots of people use tools to build things. Tina handed her dad a saw. Cindy pounded the nails in with a hammer. Brian turned the screw with a screwdriver.

Alternatives

A   Mother put flowers into the vase.

B   Susan ran to answer the phone.

C   Josh used the pliers to tighten the bolt.

24. Target Set

Grandmother's house is full of nice furniture. Tony fell asleep on grandmother's bed. We sat on the couch to watch TV. Liz did her homework at the desk.

Alternatives

A   Mary spilled milk on the rug.

B   The coffee pot is empty.

C   We had lunch at the kitchen table.

25. Target Set

We don't go to school barefoot. Ellen will put on her shoes. Jack has a hole in his sock. Mary likes to wear her new boots.

Alternatives

A **Kim has outgrown her sandals.**

B **Joe has new red gloves.**

C **The boys will play football.**

CHAPTER

9

Intervention for Advanced Literacy Skills

Principles of Advanced Literacy Intervention

1. Recognize the importance of the world knowledge children bring to the task of finding main idea and inferencing.
2. Recognize the additional processing load presented by different levels of text.
3. Use assessment results to determine where to begin.
4. Mediate for students.
5. Build on the child's existing classification and categorization abilities.

Taking a Closer Look

Principle #1: Recognize the importance of the world knowledge children bring to the task of finding the main idea and inferencing.

- Children must use their prior knowledge to engage in constructive comprehension or to see connections between details and main ideas in text.
- A child who has limited prior knowledge about particular topics found in a text will have a harder time engaging in constructive comprehension.
- In intervention activities, choose materials about which children have some prior knowledge.
- Engage the child in discussion designed to help call up prior knowledge before beginning work with a text.

Principle #2: Recognize the additional processing load presented by different levels of text.

- When children with language impairments have difficulty decoding unfamiliar vocabulary or interpreting complex sentences in the text, they are confronted with a linguistic processing load that may interfere with their ability to engage in constructive comprehension.
- In the beginning, use simple, familiar text to teach the constructive comprehension strategies.
- Once the child has grasped the strategies, move to more complex text.

Principle #3: Use assessment results to determine where to begin.

- Select assessment tools that demonstrate what a child is able to do, as well as what the child cannot do.
- If assessment tools based on text are too complex for a child, back up to pictures or single words to investigate the child's use of relevant strategies.
- Begin with all students, regardless of age, based on performance levels determined by assessment.

Principle # 4: Mediate for students.

- The connection between what they already know and comprehension of text will not be apparent to students and must be explained.
- Mediation during training gives students opportunities to see how far they have come and to continue to relate what they do in the intervention setting to what happens in the classroom.
- Working with the child in the classroom, serving as a "coach" for a comprehension task in that setting, will help the child understand the carryover from the intervention setting to the classroom.

Principle #5: Build on the child's existing classification and categorization abilities.

- Begin by explaining the relationship between basic categorization skills, which the child can demonstrate using pictures, and finding the main idea of a text.
- Begin inferencing intervention by using simple scripts for events you are sure the child has experienced, making it clear to the student that when he or she tells what the script is about, the child is doing what is needed to understand text.
- Basing intervention on abilities the child knows he or she already has will motivate the child to work harder.

Goals and Objectives for Advanced Literacy

The goals and objectives for learning advanced literacy skills focus clinicians on helping students gain meaning from written text. They are stated using educational terms for easy alignment with typical school curricula. Once again, this list should be used as a starting point when trying to formulate IEPs for students who are struggling to use language to learn advanced literacy skills.

We have begun instruction in this area with students as young as 8 years of age and as old as 17, with some students at each age level needing to begin main idea instruction with categorization, stating oral definitions, and structured conversation. Why use these skills as a foundation for instruction when beginning to teach advanced literacy skills? Experience has taught us that students with language impairment need help bridging the gap between oral and written communication skills.

Goal

The student will increase categorization and classification abilities to support development of advanced literacy skills.

Objectives

- To categorize items in a variety of ways including appearance, function, and use.
- To classify items belonging to the same category as people, places, or things.
- To name a specific category for a group of items.
- To state oral definitions using the framework, "A _____ is a _____that _____. "
- To classify main ideas and supporting details.
- To associate supporting details with a given main idea.
- To associate a main idea with a given set of supporting details.

Goal

The student will use advanced literacy skills to increase reading comprehension ability.

Objectives

- To define the term "topic" within the context of a familiar activity.
- To define the term "main idea" within the context of a familiar activity.
- To define the term "supporting details" within the context of a familiar activity.
- To state the topic of an informational paragraph.
- To state the main idea of an informational paragraph given the supporting details.
- To state the supporting details from an informational paragraph given the main idea.
- To state the main idea of an informational paragraph.
- To state the supporting details from an informational paragraph.
- To identify comprehension questions about a paragraph that require an inference.
- To use experience and world knowledge to make inferences and engage in constructive comprehension.

Goal

The student will use advanced literacy skills to increase written language ability.

Objectives

- To plan a paragraph about a topic given the "main idea."
- To plan a paragraph about a topic given three supporting details.
- To plan a paragraph about a topic that includes a main idea and three supporting details.
- To draft a paragraph about a topic given the main idea and three supporting details.
- To draft a paragraph about a topic given the main idea.
- To draft a paragraph about a topic given three supporting details.
- To draft a paragraph about a topic that includes a main idea and three supporting details.

A Word About Our Lesson Plans for Advanced Literacy Intervention

Our goal in this section is to demonstrate one way to begin organizing intervention in advanced literacy. We have developed lessons that teach strategies for giving oral definitions, identifying main ideas and supporting details, planning and drafting paragraphs about a topic, and making inferences. These provide a framework for developing advanced literacy skills with school-aged children and should be modified to meet the individual needs of students.

Our lessons for teaching main idea move from using stories as a context for intervention to using expository text. Although in classrooms across the country students are asked to tell the "main idea" of a story, recognizing and stating the "main idea" should be a task reserved for assessing comprehension of expository text. Whenever possible, the student's social studies and science textbooks should be the primary context for intervention.

Collaboration with special education and general education teachers is critical to the development of advanced literacy skills. Clinicians need to know grade-level expectations and classroom curriculum. Teachers need to know intervention strategies and the approach being used to teach them. Sharing information prepares clinicians to develop academically relevant intervention activities and helps teachers to include students with language impairment in classroom instruction and maximize their performance.

The notion of "mastery" with this type of intervention is complex. Some students may gradually understand "main idea" at a level commensurate with grade-level peers. They may successfully apply strategies to grade-level materials across a variety of contexts. For students with this potential, criteria for mastery of advanced literacy skills should be performance at grade level. For students with more complex needs, the ability to find a main idea and make inferences may never exceed third grade level.

Each lesson plan includes:

1. Introduction to procedures
2. Objectives for each lesson
3. Materials needed
4. Basic clinician role and demonstration
5. Student role
6. Suggested cueing strategies
7. Suggested criteria for mastery for each lesson

Taking a Closer Look

The **introduction** for each lesson includes a reminder of its clinical and educational relevance, which contains general information about developing targeted skills. It also may suggest certain contexts that have proven successful in our experience.

The **objectives** for each lesson are presented in simple form. They should be made measurable by the clinician or teacher by adding a context and criteria. We feel that the most important criteria is the effect intervention has on a student's abilities to perform in the classroom. Some school districts insist that progress be reported strictly in terms of percentage accuracy, others acknowledge that reporting gains in terms of the amount of support a child needs to maintain performance levels similar to those of their peers is more meaningful. A list of all the goals and objectives for advanced literacy intervention is also included.

The **materials** needed for each lesson are listed. The children's books that are listed are currently in print and should be available at a local library, bookstore, or on-line book vendor. The primary material, we feel, should be the classroom textbooks. It is in these textbooks that the child will be required to demonstrate literacy skills.

The **clinician's role** in each lesson is outlined to give clinicians, teachers, and parents a general idea of how to talk to students about these issues. It is not meant to be "the only way" to talk with students, but it should give an indication of our approach. We feel that a demonstration is a very powerful tool. With a demonstration, the clinician or teacher can help a student with language impairment more readily than with a verbal discussion or instructions. Accompany the demonstration by verbalizing your thinking strategies. It is these strategies that students need to learn. Mediation is also a powerful communication tool. Be sure that the students know the purpose of each activity and how they can use this strategy in the classroom.

The **student's role** in each lesson is provided to give clinicians, teachers, and parents an idea of what students say or do when their responses are appropriate. This section also provides suggested cues if the student does not give the expected response.

Suggested cueing strategies are described because of the importance of providing scaffolding throughout the intervention process. The cues provided are taken directly from our clinical and classroom experiences with students. They vary in nature and intensity, depending on the student's response to a given learning opportunity. If students seem to rely too heavily on cues, consider the need for additional demonstration or teaching.

Suggested criteria for mastery of specific concepts are outlined for each lesson. We generally recommend reaching a mastery level of performance before proceeding to the next lesson. However, in special cases in which mastery learning is not a realistic expectation, criteria for moving to the next lesson may need to be set on an individual basis. Under these circumstances, frequent review of previously "learned" concepts through direct practice and mediation is the key to successful intervention.

Lesson Plans for Advanced Literacy Intervention

Teaching Main Idea: Giving Oral Definitions

Introduction

Giving an oral definition for a familiar word is a metalinguistic task that serves as a building block to identifying the main idea. It gives students the opportunity to practice telling about something they know in a decontextualized manner. It requires students to name a category for an item and state the most important information that describes it. Students who cannot define familiar words orally are not ready to learn more sophisticated advanced literacy skills.

Objectives

The objectives for teaching oral definitions focus on developing underlying categorization skills as well as on using a specific framework to structure the oral definition.

Materials

A clinician-constructed copy of the definition framework large enough for all students to view is needed. In addition, a visual representation of the item to be defined should be available for students to handle.

Clinician's Role

The clinician chooses words for students to define that are familiar to them and provides a visual referent for students to use throughout the activity. The clinician steers students away from telling about personal experiences by helping them brainstorm a list of everything they know about the item. For example, a definition for the word "deer" should not include a description of a hunting experience. The word "deer" is defined as follows: "A *deer* is a *wild animal* that *lives in the woods and has huge antlers.*"

Student's Role

The students categorize the item to be defined as a person, place, or thing. If possible, a more specific category is then named, such as "food" or "animal." Then students participate in brainstorming a list of what they know about the item. Students select one or more ideas that best define the item and each uses the framework to formulate an oral definition.

Suggested Cueing Strategies

Verbal cues that support students include giving "either/or choices" and organizing brainstorming ideas into "very important" information about the item and "not important" information about the item.

Suggested Criteria for Mastery

Mastery is suggested when a student independently gives oral definitions using the framework.

Lesson Plan: Giving Oral Definitions

Objectives

1. To categorize items in a variety of ways, including appearance, function, and use.

2. To classify items belonging to the same category, such as people, places, or things.

3. To name a specific category for a group of items.

4. To state oral definitions using the framework, "A _____is a _____that _____."

Materials

- A visual representation of the item being defined. (picture or manipulative)
- A copy of the written framework for giving an oral definition.

    A _____ is a _____that _____.

Activity

The student gives an oral definition for a familiar word. A framework is used to structure the definition. The clinician teaches the student to define a word by completing the framework with a category name and the most important information about the item being defined.

Procedures

Demonstration: The clinician externalizes the thought process for naming a category, brainstorming the most important information about the item being defined, and using the framework to organize an oral definition. The clinician records the definition on a written copy of the framework.

- ○ **Clinician:** State a word to be defined and show a visual representation. Ask the students, "What is a _____?"

- ○ **Students:** Respond with the name of a category.

- ○ **Clinician:** Fill in the category name on the definition framework. Work with students to brainstorm a list of information about the item being defined. Categorize each piece of information as "important" or "not important."

- ○ **Students:** Select one or two pieces of important information that best define the item.

- ○ **Clinician:** Complete the definition by recording the most important information on the written framework. Read back to the students.

- ○ **Students:** Recite the definition.

Teaching Main Idea: Using Conversation as a Familiar Context

Introduction

We begin our instruction for main idea by using a structured conversation as a context for identifying the topic, main idea, and supporting details. We use this context because it is familiar. Students learn to state something that they can talk about for at least 5 minutes (the topic), identify the most important idea discussed about the topic (main idea), and list at least three little ideas that go with the important idea about the topic (supporting details).

Objectives

The objectives focus on developing a working knowledge of the terms "topic," "main idea," and "supporting details." These definitions should be internalized, so that students are not adding to their processing load as they attempt to understand expository text.

Materials

The only materials needed are blank main idea outlines. If students can't think of topics to talk about, any form of expository text about a familiar topic may be used. However, brainstorming a list of topics with the clinician is a better option for this lesson.

Clinician's Role

The clinician's role is, through commentary, to keep the conversation moving and on track, using the terms topic, main idea, and supporting details. For example, if the students decide to talk about basketball and someone starts talking about soccer, the clinician says, "You can't talk about soccer right now because we decided that the *topic* of our conversation is basketball." Another example is, "Our conversation is full of *details* about kids getting injured while playing basketball, so I guess the *main idea* is that basketball can be a dangerous sport." The clinician demonstrates how to record the analysis of the structured conversation on a main idea outline.

Student's Role

The student's role at this stage is to actively participate in the structured conversation. The student must think of topics to talk about and stick with them. The student also needs to practice stating definitions for the terms *topic*, *main idea*, and *supporting details.*

Suggested Cueing Strategies

The clinician cues students by using the terms and their definitions within the context of the structured conversation. For example, "Wait a minute Billy you just changed the *topic*, we agreed to only talk about basketball for now." Another helpful cueing strategy is the open-ended sentence. For example, "I heard a lot of talking about '_____.'" That seems to be *the most important idea* about our *topic*.

Suggested Criteria for Mastery

Criteria for mastery is the ability to give working definitions of the terms *topic*, *main idea*, and *supporting details* and consistently identify them in a structured conversation.

Lesson Plan: Teaching Main Idea Through Conversation

Objectives

1. To define the term "topic" within the context of a familiar activity.
2. To define the term "main idea" within the context of a familiar activity.
3. To define the term "details" within the context of a familiar activity.

Materials

- Main idea outline (an example follows this lesson plan).
- A list of topics students can talk about.
- Expository text (use text that the students are using in the classroom).

Activity

Students state a topic that they can talk about for at least 5 minutes. The clinician listens to the conversation and comments on the main idea as it emerges. The topic, main idea, and supporting details from the conversation are recorded on a simple outline provided by the clinician. Gradually, the students take over the role of analyzing the conversation and recording the topic, main idea, and supporting details in outline form.

Procedure

Demonstration: Mediate for students. Explain the importance of understanding what one reads by determining the topic, main idea and supporting details. Discuss and define the terms "topic," "main idea," and "details" as simply as possible. Explain that learning to find the main idea can be confusing and that practicing the skill during conversation is often helpful.

- A "topic" is something people can talk about.
- A "main idea" is the most important idea about the topic
- A "detail" is a little idea that supports (goes with) the main idea about the topic.

  - ○ **Clinician:** Ask the students to name three things they like to do (i.e., play basketball, go to movies, ride horses). Explain that each is a topic. Ask the students to choose one of these topics and talk about it in a conversation for 5–10 minutes. It may be necessary to mediate occasionally to be sure that the students stay on topic and that everyone gets equal opportunity.

  - ○ **Students:** Talk among themselves and with the clinician about the chosen topic.

  - ○ **Clinician:** Takes notes of the main ideas and supporting details that the students express during the conversation.

  - ○ **Students:** Make a list of the main ideas from the conversation through discussion with the clinician.

  - ○ **Students:** Make a list of the details taken from the conversation that support the main idea through discussion with the clinician.

  - ○ **Students:** Record the topic, main idea, and three details from the conversation on a main idea outline.

Main Idea Outline

Topic: _____

Main Idea: _____

_____

_____

Details:

1. _____

_____

_____

2. _____

_____

_____

3. _____

_____

_____

Notes:

Teaching Main Idea: A Classification Task

Introduction

Now that students can give oral definitions for familiar vocabulary and have developed a working knowledge of the terms *topic, main idea,* and *supporting details,* they are ready for the next step. Using a classification task, students learn to sort written sentences into the categories of *main idea sentences* and *detail sentences.* Once sorted, students are instructed to determine which *details* are associated with a given *main idea.*

Objectives

The objectives for this lesson apply classification and categorization skills to the main idea task. They build on earlier work in defining familiar vocabulary. Students need to decide which sentences state *details* and which sentences state *main ideas.*

Materials

Because the concept of main idea is a function of expository text, the materials we use for teaching main idea strategies are social studies and science textbooks, newspaper articles, and magazine articles. At least two or three passages from a source are retyped on separate sheets of paper and cut into strips for ease of sorting.

Clinician's Role

The clinician's role is to support students by externalizing the thinking process used to sort *main idea* sentences from *detail* sentences. The materials selected by the clinician are also important. They should cover topics familiar to students and written at an appropriate reading level, if at all possible. Ideally, grade level texts should eventually be used.

Student's Role

The student's role is to stay positive about learning this challenging task. Students need to value reading comprehension skills and recognize that being able to find the main idea is critical for school success. They should be actively involved in discussion of a topic and the identification and organization of a main idea and supporting details.

Suggested Cueing Strategies

We cue students by reminding them of our working definitions for the terms *main idea* and *supporting details.* We give them thinking strategies such as, "Read the sentence strip again. Does the idea sound like a *big* one or a *little* one that goes with a *big* one?" Our sentence frame cue works well when students struggle associating the right details with a given main idea. For example, "This detail about how lions tear food with their teeth goes with the main idea about how lions _____."

Suggested Criteria for Mastery

Students should independently classify sentences as *main ideas* or *supporting details* using the format, "These are all _____." Then they should accurately associate at least three details with each main idea.

Lesson Plan: Teaching Main Idea Through Classification

Objectives

1. To classify "main ideas" and "details."
2. To associate "details" with a given "main idea."
3. To associate a "main idea" with a given set of "details."

Materials

- Children's books that contain expository text about a topic. (We use books by Seymour Simon such as *Big Cats* and *Storms*.)
- Three sentence strips with main ideas.
- Three sets of sentence strips with supporting details (1 set for each main idea).

Activity

Students classify sentences as stating *main ideas* or *supporting details*. Once classified, they use each main idea sentence as a category and sort the supporting details so that they go with the appropriate main idea sentence. At the end of the activity, students have matched all sentence strips with supporting details to a main idea sentence.

Procedures

Demonstration: Mediate for students. Remind students that when teachers ask, "What is the most important idea about what you have read?" they are asking, "What is the main idea?"

Select a book or magazine article about a topic familiar to students. Select a paragraph with a clearly stated main idea and at least three supporting details. Show students the paragraph typed as a list of sentences. Cut the list into sentence strips. Mix up the sentence strips. Find the sentence that states the main idea by comparing the sentences. Talk through the process of identifying the main idea by referring to the definition of main idea. Explain that the remaining sentences strips tell details that support the main idea.

     ○ **Clinician:** Select three new paragraphs with clearly stated main ideas. Type the sentences that make up each paragraph into lists. Cut each list into sentence strips. Keep the sentence strips for each paragraph together.

Read one of the paragraphs aloud. Give the students the sentence strips that go with the paragraph, and ask them to try and find the main idea sentence. Encourage students to refer back to the text as necessary.

Note: We are teaching the student a strategy for comprehending text. We are not working on the child's memory for text.

- ○ **Student:** Find the sentence strip that tells the main idea by recalling the definition of main idea stated earlier.

- ○ **Clinician:** Repeat the same procedure with the other two paragraphs.

- ○ **Clinician:** Spread out the three "main idea" sentences (one for each paragraph) the students have found in one area. Mix up the "supporting detail" sentences and spread them out in another location. Tell students to physically match the "supporting detail" sentences to the appropriate "main idea" sentence.

- ○ **Student:** Sort the supporting detail sentences using the main idea sentences as categories.

- ○ **Clinician:** Give students the three "main idea" sentences. Mix together the "detail" sentences from all three paragraphs.

Note: It is important to mediate throughout each step. Require students to explain their decisions using the terms "topic," "main idea," and "details."

Teaching Main Idea: Strategies for Reading Comprehension and Expository Writing

Introduction

Students with language impairment need clinicians to break down the task of finding the main idea and provide them with strategies for approaching the task one step at a time. The following lessons are designed to teach students with language impairment about main idea at the paragraph level by making sure they can differentiate between main idea sentences and those that state supporting details. Students are taught to use a simple outlining strategy for both taking a paragraph apart and drafting a paragraph about a familiar topic.

Objectives

The objectives for using advanced literacy skills to increase reading comprehension and written language ability are in alignment with most middle elementary school curricula. They can be made measurable by adding a context, or performance level, or stating that the student will complete tasks provided with a specific level of support by the clinician.

Materials

Children's books containing expository writing about familiar topics are used as a context for teaching about main idea. Main idea outlines are preprinted by the clinician and made available to students for both comprehension and written expression tasks.

Clinician's Role

The clinician should select materials with which students can experience success. For one student this may involve using materials that support classroom curricula, but are easier to read and understand than grade-level text. For another, the clinician may need to simplify the main idea task by using materials appropriate to the student's world knowledge.

Student's Role

The student plays an active role through discussion, note taking, reading, and writing.

Suggested Cueing Strategies

We use two basic cueing strategies if a student has difficulty responding appropriately for the remaining main idea lessons. First, we direct the student on where to look in a paragraph. Although in most well-written elementary material, the main idea will be in the first sentence, we do not want to teach the student that the main idea is always the first sentence. Second, we tell the child the supporting details in the paragraph and see if he or she can identify the main idea from them. Try the sentence frame, "These little ideas are all about _____."

Suggested Criteria for Mastery

When the student can identify the main idea when explicitly stated in grade-level material, intervention should shift to identifying the main idea when implied in text.

Criteria for mastery should be reading comprehension using grade-level materials.

Lesson Plan: Identifying and Writing Supporting Details

Objectives

1. To state the "supporting details" from an informational paragraph given the "main idea."
2. To plan a paragraph about a topic given the "main idea."
3. To draft a paragraph about a topic given the "main idea."

Materials

- Children's books that contain expository text about a topic. (We use books by Seymour Simon such as *Big Cats* and *Storms* or passages from children's magazines.)
- Main idea outlines

Activity

Students are given the opportunity to listen to a paragraph read aloud by the clinician as they follow along. They are told the main idea, but are asked to select key words that represent details from the paragraph. They record the key words as "notes" and later use them to formulate sentences. They use the "detail" sentences to complete the main idea outline.

Procedure

Demonstration: Show a book or magazine article about a topic familiar to the students. Read the paragraph aloud as students follow along. Tell the main idea of the paragraph and write it on the outline. Read the paragraph aloud again. Show them how to listen for key words that signal details that support the main idea.

- ○ **Clinician:** Read another paragraph. Instruct students to listen and write down key words that signal details about the main idea.

- ○ **Students:** Write down key words in the "Notes" section of the main idea outline.

- ○ **Clinician:** Demonstrate taking a key word and turning it into a sentence that tells a supporting detail for the main idea.

- ○ **Students:** Construct at least three detail sentences using their key words and write the sentences on a main idea outline.

- ○ **Clinician:** Check the sentences to make sure they are complete and tell details that support the main idea.

- ○ **Students:** Use the main idea outline as a plan for drafting a paragraph with a main idea and at least 3 supporting details.

Note: It is important to mediate throughout each step. Require students to explain their decisions using the terms "topic," "main idea," and "details."

Lesson Plan: Identifying and Writing Main Ideas

Objectives

1. To state the "main idea" of a paragraph given the "supporting "details."
2. To plan a paragraph about a topic given three supporting details.
3. To draft a paragraph about a topic given three supporting details.

Materials

- Children's books that contain expository text about a topic. (We use books by Seymour Simon such as *Big Cats* and *Storms* or passages from children's magazines.)
- Main idea outlines

Activity

Students are given the opportunity to listen to a paragraph read aloud by the clinician as they follow along. They are told the supporting details, but are asked to determine the main idea of the paragraph. They are cued to determine the topic and are then to ask themselves, "What is the most important idea about the topic?" They are cued to refer to the details to help them answer this question. They state the main idea in sentence form and complete the main idea outline. They use the outline as a "plan" for drafting a paragraph.

Procedures

Demonstration: Show a book or magazine article about a topic familiar to the students. Show a paragraph with a clearly stated main idea and supporting details. Read the paragraph aloud as students follow along. Tell the details that support the main idea of the paragraph and show them written as sentences on the outline. Read the paragraph aloud again. Show them how to complete three sentence frames as a strategy for finding the main idea of the paragraph.

○ **Clinician:** Select a book or magazine article about a topic familiar to the students. Select a paragraph with a clearly stated "main idea" and "details." Provide a main idea outline with the "supporting details" stated. Read the entire paragraph aloud.

○ **Students:** Read the details stated on the outline and determine the main idea by completing the following sentence frames:

- The topic of the paragraph is _____.
- The details in the paragraph tell all about _____.
- Since the details in a paragraph tell all about the main idea, the main idea must be _____.

○ **Clinician:** Help students complete the sentence frames.

Note: If the students have difficulty with this type of task it may be necessary to do more work with the classification of details and main ideas and the relationship between the two.

○ **Students:** Complete the main idea outline by filling in a sentence that tells about the main idea.

○ **Clinician:** Review the completed outline with the students and demonstrate how to use it as a plan for drafting a paragraph.

○ **Students:** Draft a paragraph using the main idea outline as a guide.

Lesson Plan: Identifying the Main Idea and Supporting Details

Objectives

1. To state the main idea and supporting details of an informational paragraph read or heard.

2. To plan a paragraph about a topic that includes a main idea and three supporting details.

3. To draft a paragraph about a topic that includes a main idea and three supporting details.

Materials

- Children's books that contain expository text about a topic. (We use books by Seymour Simon such as *Big Cats* and *Storms* or passages from children's magazines.)
- Main idea outlines

Activity

Students have the opportunity to complete a main idea outline by identifying both the main idea and supporting details from a paragraph, then use it as a plan for drafting a paragraph about the topic they read about.

Procedures

- **Clinician:** Select a book or magazine article about a topic familiar to the students. Select a paragraph with a clearly stated "main idea" and clear "details." Provide a blank copy of a "main idea" outline. Read the entire paragraph aloud as the students follow along.

- **Students:** Students independently complete the "main idea" outline using the key word strategy and the sentence frame strategy, making a plan for drafting a paragraph about a topic.

- **Clinician:** Review the plan with the students to be sure the details and the main idea make sense.

- **Students:** Draft a paragraph using the main idea outline as a plan.

- **Clinician:** The clinician notes any areas of difficulty and returns to previous lessons if needed.

Teaching Inferencing and Constructive Comprehension

Introduction

One major aspect of reading comprehension in the upper elementary grades and beyond is inferencing. Making predictions and drawing conclusions are based on the ability to infer meaning. To make an inference, one needs to apply past experiences and knowledge, as well as the facts from the text. Many students with language-impairment are very literal thinkers. If a teacher asks a question about the text, a student with language impairment frequently assumes that he or she is supposed to find the answer in the text. They frequently approach each text encounter as if it is the first time they have ever heard anything about a subject.

Objectives

In teaching students who are language impaired about inferencing, the goal should be to help them organize their ideas so that they can access both "new" and "old" information. To do this, it is necessary that a student learn to recognize when a question is asking for inferencing. Further, it is necessary for the student to recognize what he or she already knows about the topic. In this vein, objectives are directed toward teaching the semantic cues that signal an inferencing question and making and using a prepartory set of known information to draw from.

Materials

Whenever possible the materials for these lessons should come from the student's classroom. A child needs to learn to apply these skills to his or her own textbooks. The best way for a student to learn to use a skill in a particular environment is to teach him the skill in that environment.

Clinician's Role

The clinician's role is to provide opportunities for a student to learn strategies for answering inferencing questions. The clinician should provide materials appropriate to a student's world experience. It is easier to deal with inferencing questions when reading about a subject with which you have some experience. The clinician must provide demonstration and externalize the thinking process for the student. Continual review of the strategies employed to identify and answer inferencing questions will assure that the student retains a skill.

Student's Role

The student should be actively involved in the discussion of the topic and the identification and answering of inferencing questions.

Suggested Cueing Strategies

If the student has difficulty with the inferencing question provide a cue such as:

1. Changing the question to a fill-in the blank question (i.e., instead of "Why did he take a pole and worms with him?" Change it to "He took a pole and worms because _____").

2. Ask the child to put him- or herself in that situation "Why would you _____?"

3. Refer back to the list the student made of things he or she already knows about the subject,

4. Have the student state the main idea of the section he or she just read.

Suggested Criteria for Mastery

The suggested criterion for mastery that is the most relevant is the teacher's judgment of a student's reading comprehension abilities. If the student can answer inferencing questions using grade level materials, then mastery is suggested.

Lesson Plan: Identifying Inferencing Questions

Objective

To identify questions that require inferencing.

Materials

- Clinician-constructed paragraphs based on topics familiar to the students.
- Clinician-constructed literal and inferential comprehension questions based on the example paragraph.
- Paragraphs and comprehension questions from the student's classroom materials, including social studies and science textbooks.

Activity

The activities are designed to help a child recognize that the student already has information about the topic he or she is reading. The activities teach the child to bring that prior information to the foreground (preparatory set). The activities teach the child to recognize the signal that the question requires inferencing.

Procedure

Demonstration: Inferencing activities are most appropriate when inferencing becomes a major aspect of text comprehension—generally third grade and above. Mediation should include a statement that teachers always ask questions about what students read. Sometimes the answers to the questions are on the page. Sometimes they are not on the page. It is important to know whether an answer is on the page or not. It is important to know how to answer the question, if the answer is not on the page.

> **Example paragraph:** It is John's job to bring home something for his family to eat. In the morning he took his pole and worms to the river. Later that day he came home with five fish.

> Who is in this story?

> What time of day was it?

> Where did he go?

> Why did he take a pole and worms with him?

> How do you think he felt when he came home?

> - **Clinician:** Discuss the topic of the prepared paragraph with the child making a list of everything he or she knows about the topic (fishing).

> - **Student:** Lists everything he or she knows about fishing.

> - **Clinician:** Read or have the child read the paragraph and questions. Ask the child to answer each question. Ask the child how he or she knew the answer (found the answer in the text or "thought it up").

> - **Student:** Reads the paragraph and answers the questions. If the student has difficulty with the inferencing questions, refer the child back to the list made of everything he or she knows about fishing.

> - **Clinician:** Present two or three similarly constructed paragraphs and questions. Ask the child to identify (highlight) the questions that he or she knew the answers to because of his previous experience. Ask the stu-

dent to look at the words used in those questions. What are used in those questions but not in the others?

- ○ **Student:** Highlights the inferencing questions and identifies that they use words like "why" and "you think."

- ○ **Clinician:** Using the student's textbook, select a section already studied in class. Turn to the end of the section and ask the child to read the questions and choose which ones to ask him or her to answer from personal knowledge.

- ○ **Student:** Identifies the inferencing questions. Point out that the child's textbook calls some questions "Thinking Questions." When students see this phrase, they know they need to think of an answer from information they already have.

Note: Many children with language impairment are very literal. They expect that an answer to every question should be found in the text. Part of what SLPs need to make explicit for them is that they can and must use what they already know about a subject to answer some of the questions.

Lesson Plan: Answering Inferencing Questions

Objective

Use previous experience and world knowledge to make inferences and engage in constructive comprehension.

Materials

- Content are texts, especially social studies.
- Questions to be answered by students

Activity

After the student can distinguish an inferencing question, the SLP should provide strategies that the child can use to answer the inferencing question. Although the classroom textbook is used, the course content is not being taught.

Procedures

Demonstration: Engage the student in a conversation about the topic of the segment of text that you will be using in intervention. Help the child make a list of everything he or she already knows about this topic. Tell the child that, as he answers the "thinking questions" at the end of the chapter, he can refer to this list.

- ○ **Clinician:** Remind the student that you are working on learning how to answer questions about things the child has read. Tell the child that sometimes it is helpful to turn to the back of the chapter to read the questions first, so he or she can think about them while reading. Ask the student to read the questions and decide which ones are inferencing questions ("thinking questions").

○ **Student:** Reads and classifies the questions.

○ **Clinician:** Have the child read the section of text and answer the first inferencing question ("thinking question"). Be sure to ask the student how he or she knew that answer.

○ **Student:** Answers questions from the text. If the student has difficulty with this task, refer to the cueing suggestions.

○ **Clinician:** After several successful examples, review for the student the strategies that helped him or her answer the questions.

1. Read the paragraph heading and make a list of everything you know about the topic.

2. Turn to the back of the section and read the questions. Decide which ones are "thinking questions."

3. Read the section with the "thinking questions" in mind.

4. If you are not sure how to answer the "thinking question," change it into a fill-in-the-blank question or think of the things you already know about the topic, or think what you would do if you were the person in the text.

Note: Some teachers may think that looking at questions before reading the section is "cheating." However, most good students learn to do this without being taught. Looking ahead to the questions is another way to help a child with language impairment lessen the processing load. The student can learn to answer the questions as he or she goes along so that it is not necessary to remember everything. It also makes the process less overwhelming to the student.

References

Anderson, R. (1994). Role of the reader's schemata in comprehension, Learning and memory. In R. B. Ruddell, M. Rapp, & H. Singers (Eds.), *Theoretical models and processes of reading* (4th ed., pp. 469–482). Newark, DE: International Reading Association.

Ball, E., & Blachman, B. (1991). Does phoneme awareness training in kindergarten make a difference in early word recognition and developmental spelling? *Reading Research Quarterly, 26,* 49–66.

Baumann, J. (1984). The effectiveness of a direct instruction paradigm for teaching main idea comprehension. *Reading Research Quarterly, 20,* 93–105.

Baumann, J. (1986). The direct instruction of main idea comprehension ability. In J. Baumann (Ed.), *Teaching main idea comprehension* (pp. 133–193). Newark, DE: International Reading Association.

Bishop, D., & Adams, C. (1990). A prospective study of the relationship between specific language impairment, phonological disorders and reading retardation. *Journal of Child Psychology and Psychiatry, 31,* 1027–1050.

Blachman, B. (1991). Early intervention for children's reading problems: Clinical applications of the research in phonological awareness. *Topics in Language Disorders, 12,* 51–65.

Blachman, B. (1994). Language analysis skills and early reading acquisition. In G. Wallach & K. Butler (Eds.), *Language learning disabilities in school-age children* (pp. 271–287). Baltimore, MD: Williams & Wilkins.

Blachman, B., Ball, E., Black, S., & Tangel, D. (1994). Kindergarten teachers develop phoneme awareness in low-income, inner-city classrooms: Does it make a difference? *Reading and Writing: An Interdisciplinary Journal, 6,* 1–17.

Blachowicz, C. (1994). Problem-solving strategies for academic success. In G. Wallach & K. Butler (Eds.), *Language learning disabilities in school-age children* (pp. 253–274). Baltimore, MD: Williams & Wilkins.

Bradley, L., & Bryant, P. (1983). Categorizing sounds and learning to read: A causal connection. *Nature, 301,* 419–421.

Bradley, L., & Bryant, P. (1985). *Rhyme and reason in reading and spelling.* (International Academy for Research in Learning Disabilities Monograph Series, No. 1.) Ann Arbor: University of Michigan Press.

Catts, H. (1989). Phonological processing deficits and reading disabilities. In A. Kamhi & H. Catts (Eds.), *Reading disabilities: A developmental language perspective.* Boston: Allyn & Bacon.

Catts, H. (1993). The relationship between speech-language impairments and reading disabilities. *Journal of Speech and Hearing Research, 36,* 948–958.

Catts, H., & Kamhi, A. (Eds.). (1998). *Language and reading disabilities.* Needham Heights, MA: Allyn & Bacon.

Crais, E., & Chapman, R. (1987). Story recall and inferencing skills in language learning disabled and nondisabled children. *Journal of Speech and Hearing Disorders, 52,* 50–55.

Ellis Weismer, S. (1985). Constructive comprehension abilities exhibited by language-disordered children. *Journal of Speech and Hearing Research, 28,* 175–184.

Fazio, B., Naremore, R., & Connell, P. (1996). Tracking children from poverty at risk for specific language impairment: A 3-year longitudinal study. *Journal of Speech and Hearing Research, 39,* 611–624.

Fletcher, J., Shaywitz, S. Shankweiler, D., Katz, L., Liberman, I., Stuebing, K., Francis, D., Fowler, A., & Shaywitz, B. (1994). Cognitive profiles of reading disability: Comparisons of discrepancy and low achievement definitions. *Journal of Educational Psychology, 86,* 6–23.

Gillam, R., McFadden, T., & van Kleek, A. (1995). Improving the narrative abilities of children with language disorders: Whole language and language skills approaches. In M. Fey, J. Windsor, & S. Warren (Eds.), *Language intervention: Preschool through the elementary years.* Baltimore, MD: Paul H. Brookes.

Graham, S., MacArthur, C., Schwartz, S., & Voth, T. (1992). Improving the compositions of students with learning disabilities using a strategy involving product and process goal setting. *Exceptional Children, 58,* 322–335.

Hansen, C. (1978). Story retelling used with average and learning disabled readers as a measure of reading comprehension. *Learning Disability Quarterly, 1,* 62–69.

Hansen, J., & Pearson, P. (1983). An instructional study: Improving the inferential comprehension of good and poor fourth grade readers. *Journal of Educational Psychology, 75,* 821–829.

Hatcher, P., Hulme, C., & Ellis, A. (1994). Ameliorating early reading failure by integrating the teaching of reading and phonological skills: The phonological linkage hypothesis. *Child Development, 65,* 41–57.

Hudson, J., & Nelson, K. (1983). Effects of script structure on children's story recall. *Developmental Psychology, 19,* 625–635.

Hudson, J., & Shapiro. L. (1991). From knowing to telling: The development of children's scripts, stories, and personal narratives. In A. McCabe & C. Peterson (Eds.), *Developing narrative structure* (pp. 89–136). Hillsdale, NJ: Erlbaum.

Kamhi, A., & Catts, H. (1986). Toward an understanding of developmental language and reading disorders. *Journal of Speech and Hearing Disorders, 51,* 337–347.

Klecan-Aker, J., & Caraway, T. (1997). A study of the relationship of storytelling ability to reading comprehension in fourth and sixth grade African-American children. *European Journal of Disorders of Communication, 32,* 109–125.

Lahey, M., & Bloom, L. (1994). Variability and language learning disabilities. In G. Wallach & K. Butler (Eds.), *Language learning disabilities in school-age children and adolescents* (pp. 354–372). New York: Merrill.

Liberman, I., & Shankweiler, D. (1985). Phonology and the problems of learning to read and write. *Remedial and Special Education, 6,* 8–17.

Liberman, I., & Shankweiler, D. (1991). Phonology and beginning reading: A tutorial. In L. Rieben & C. Perfetti (Eds.), *Learning to read: Basic research and its implications.* Hillsdale, NJ: Erlbaum.

Liles, B., Duffy, R., Merritt, D., & Purcell, S. (1995). Measurement of narrative discourse ability in children with language disorders. *Journal of Speech and Hearing Research, 38,* 415–425.

Lundberg, I., Frost, J., & Petersen, O. (1988). Effects of an extensive program for stimulating phonological awareness in preschool children. *Reading Research Quarterly, 23,* 264–284.

Mann, V. A. (1993). Phoneme awareness and future reading ability. *Journal of Learning Disabilities, 26,* 259–269.

McCabe, A., & Rollins, P. (1994). Assessment of preschool narrative skills. *American Journal of Speech Language Pathology, 3,* 45–55.

McCauley, R. (1996). Familiar strangers: Criterion-referenced measures in communication disorders. *Language, Speech, and Hearing Services in Schools, 27,*122–131.

Naremore, R. (1997). Making it hang together: Children's use of mental frameworks to structure narratives. *Topics in Language Disorders, 18,* 16–31.

Naremore, R., Densmore, A., & Harman, D. (1995). *Language intervention with school-aged children.* San Diego, CA: Singular Publishing Group.

Nelson, K., & Greundel, J. (1986). Children's scripts. In K. Nelson (Ed.), *Event knowledge: Structure and function in development* (pp. 21–46). Hillsdale, NJ: Erlbaum.

Palinscar, A., & Brown, A. (1984). Reciprocal teaching of comprehension-fostering and comprehension-monitoring activities. *Cognition and Instruction, 1,* 117–175.

Raphael, T. E., (1982). Question answering strategies for children. *Reading Teacher, 36,* 186–190.

Roller, C. M., & Schreiner, R. (1985). The effects of narrative and expository organization instruction on sixth-grade children's comprehension of expository and narrative prose. *Reading Psychology, 6,* 27–42.

Sawyer, R., Graham, S., & Harris, K. (1992). Direct teaching, strategy instruction, and strategy instruction with explicit self-regulation: Effects on learning disabled students' compositions and self-efficacy. *Journal of Educational Psychology, 84,* 340–352.

Scott, C. M. (1989). Problem writers: Nature, assessment, and intervention. In A. Kamhi & H. Catts (Eds.), *Reading disabilities: A developmental language perspective.* Boston: Little, Brown.

Sentell, C., & Blachowicz, C. (1989) Comprehension court: A process approach to inference instruction. *The Reading Teacher, 43,* 347–348.

Stahl, S., & Murray, B. (1994). Defining phonological awareness and its relationship to early reading. *Journal of Educational Psychology, 86,* 221–234.

Taylor, M., & Williams, J. (1983). Comprehension of learning-disabled readers: Task and text variations. *Journal of Educational Psychology, 75,* 743–751.

Wallach, G. (1990). Magic buries Celtics: Looking for broader interpretations of language learning and literacy. *Topics in Language Disorders, 10,* 63–80.

Wallach, G., & Butler, K. (1994) Creating communication, literacy, and academic success. In G. Wallach & K. Butler (Eds.), *Language learning disabilities in school-age children and adolescents* (pp. 2–26). New York: Merrill.

Westby, C. (1998). Assessing and facilitating text comprehension problems. In H. Catts & A. Kamhi (Eds.), *Language and reading disabilities* (pp. 154–223). Needham Heights, MA: Allyn & Bacon.

Williams, J. (1984). Categorization, macrostructure, and finding the main idea. *Journal of Educational Psychology, 76,* 874–879.

Williams, J., Taylor, M., & Ganger, E. (1981). Text variations at the level of the individual sentences and the comprehension of simple expository paragraphs. *Journal of Educational Pscyhology, 73,* 851–865.

Wong, B. (1982). Strategic behaviors in selecting retrieval cues in gifted, normal achieving, and learning disabled children. *Journal of Learning Disabilities, 15,* 33–37.